Tai Chi Chuan
Decoding the Classics for the Modern Martial Artist

Dan Docherty

Foreword by Dr Alexandra E. Ryan

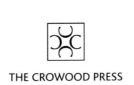

THE CROWOOD PRESS

First published in 2009 by
The Crowood Press Ltd
Ramsbury, Marlborough
Wiltshire SN8 2HR

www.crowood.com

British Library Cataloguing-in-Publication Data
A catalogue record for this book is available from the British Library.

ISBN 978 1 84797 084 8

Illustration Acknowledgements
Claire Sheehy, of University College, Dublin, took all of the action
photographs contained in this book and Birgit Müller, of the University
of Aachen, prepared all of the illustrations and diagrams.

Disclaimer
Please note that the author and the publisher of this book are not
responsible in any manner whatsoever for any damage or injury of any
kind that may result from practising, or applying, the principles, ideas,
techniques and/or following the instructions/information described in
this publication. Since the physical activities described in this book may
be too strenuous in nature for some readers to engage in safely, it is
essential that a doctor be consulted before undertaking training.

Typeset by Bookcraft, Stroud, Gloucestershire

Printed and bound in Singapore by Craft Print International Ltd

Tai Chi Chuan
Decoding the Classics for the Modern Martial Artist

圖功坐節月九露寒

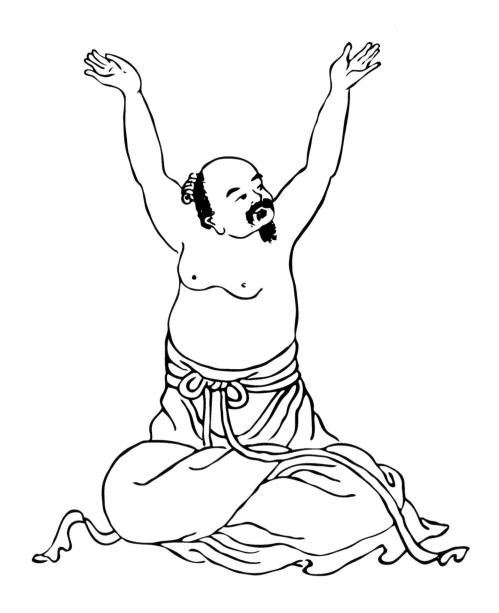

Contents

Foreword

Arguably, the more we know, the more we become aware of our differences – and the idea of universal principles seems to fade. Yet there are universals that we share – the reasons we find ourselves in conflict, or the ways we negotiate these conflicts within and between us. Chinese martial arts have something to say on these matters, and this book is part of the conversation. Its significant achievement is its original translations together with practical commentaries on the Tai Chi Chuan Classics, which illuminate both martial and meditative aspects of Tai Chi Chuan, in terms of their philosophical connections and practical manifestations.

Its secondary aim is to bring into dialogue two sets of materials: the manuals of a particular martial art – the Tai Chi Chuan Classics – and a source from the history of Chinese martial arts in general – the *Classic of Boxing*. This invites us to consider what is common and universal in martial arts. Yet the book has a deeper purpose: it provokes reflection on the interplay between philosophy and practice. Tai Chi Chuan has not always been known as a practical martial art, but it has always been known for its philosophy. On the one hand, this book separates the two spheres by juxtaposing the practical *Classic of Boxing* with the philosophical *Tai Chi Diagram* text. On the other hand, it shows connections between the two spheres within Tai Chi Chuan.

To my knowledge this is the first book in English to bring these materials together and with fresh translations as well as practical commentaries. It stands as a unique contribution to the martial arts literature, and contains a number of potential adventures for the reader. Experienced martial artists will find plenty to contemplate and debate, to test and refine, in relation to their own expertise. Beginners will no doubt find these materials inspiring and enticing. Scholars can digest a set of translations prepared by someone with practical expertise, who knows what this art is designed to do. Those like myself who have practised Tai Chi Chuan for some time, will find new stories and illustrations of the wider cultural context, fresh perspectives on the Tai Chi Chuan Classics, and undoubtedly insights into the techniques and skills of Tai Chi Chuan. I hope the readership will extend widely within and beyond the Tai Chi Chuan and martial arts communities.

Such a book could only have been written by a special author – someone unusual enough to take on this curious challenge. An endeavour like this requires expertise in Chinese language and in the cultural background, to translate the texts. It also requires extensive experience of practising and teaching Tai Chi Chuan, to produce the commentaries. Perhaps most importantly, it requires strength of will and great focus to create a book on such complex materials and do them justice. I first met Dan Docherty in 2001, when I interviewed him for my PhD research on Tai Chi Chuan in Britain. Dan embraces the polarities that run through this book, and he knows the value of developing the critical faculties as well as the skilful outer shell. He is also the only person I know who has all the ingredients within him to have been able to create this particular delicacy.

This book speaks to the idea that the interplay between our practical and philosophical aspects is the source of our greatest capabilities. In my view, that is a universal principle worth promoting.

Dr Alexandra E. Ryan

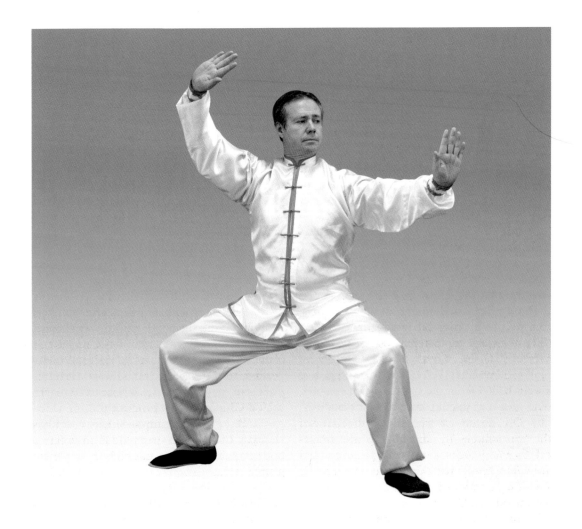

Author demonstrates Fan through the Back.

Dedication

I'd like to dedicate the book to my old comrades in the Royal Hong Kong Police.

Acknowledgements

I had a lot of help from many good people over many years in refining the material in this book. A roll of honour is published on my website, and apologies to anyone missed out.

My main assistants were a latter-day 'Three Graces': Claire Sheehy from University College Dublin, who took the action photos; Birgit Müller from the University of Aachen, who prepared the illustrations and diagrams; and Dr Alex Ryan from the University of Gloucestershire who did most of the proof-reading and advised on the structure. On the Chinese side of things, the late Cheng Tin-hung and Chen Jing-zu helped with the Tai Chi Chuan Classics, while Xin Ran gave useful suggestions on the *Classic of Boxing*.

It was good to work with Paul Mitchell, Niall Keane, Edward Connell and Alan Martin from University College Dublin, and Charles Gorrie from Glasgow, as the models for the techniques, and with Otmar Vigl and Nigel Rozier who did the action photos with me.

This book is written for the legendary 'man on the Clapham omnibus', who may practise martial arts, but almost certainly does not read Chinese. Those wishing to refer to the original Chinese texts on which my translations are based can visit my website. I have used original Chinese terms and explained them, often with a photo-graph, because many current English trans-lations are misleading. In the main I have used modern *Pinyin* romanization, except-ing well known romanizations such as Lao Tzu. I have rendered Tai Chi Chuan as TCC throughout.

Introduction

This book is for anyone practising any martial art. Its aim is to decode the theory contained in major Chinese martial arts classics so that practitioners of any martial art can understand it and do it. Those expecting an academic work will be disappointed, though much of the material is deep and subtle. The colourful cast of characters includes scholars, philosophers, Chinese emperors, martial arts instructors, Buddhist monks, Samurai warriors, itinerant Taoists and a Chinese general. The theme of duality, of Yin and Yang, of the cultural and the martial, runs through the book. It is a book about martial arts and not about 'fighting'. Pure fighting has no spiritual, therapeutic or aesthetic qualities. Martial arts are a combination of the duality of *Wen* (cultural) and *Wu* (martial), and possess all these qualities and more.

The journey is as important as the destination, and many readers may not be entirely familiar with the martial, cultural and philosophical background to the material. Part I examines what is meant by the term 'Chinese martial arts', followed by a look at the cultural background in which these arts were practised. Next comes a brief overview of the philosophical origins of Tai Chi Chuan (TCC) theory. There follows a discussion of the relationship between TCC practices and those of Taoist Internal Alchemy and meditation. Lastly we explore 'Classics' in Chinese culture.

This book presents the first fully illustrated translation and commentary on the TCC Classics. It explains to the general martial arts reader how to put the concepts of the Classics into their own practice. It is of particular use to TCC practitioners of whatever style. Part II, the core of the book, deals with this material. Many classical Chinese texts are mnemonic – designed to be chanted – and are therefore originally part of an oral tradition. This is also true of the TCC Classics. There are translations on the market already, but they are largely unsatisfactory, being written mainly by people who have little or no practical experience, and limited technical knowledge.

There is much debate about the origins of, and influences on, TCC in its early development, but there is no dispute that the *Tai Chi Diagram Explanation* and the *Classic of Boxing* did play a role in its development. Part III reproduces both texts in full, with introductions and brief commentaries to help the reader deconstruct the earlier TCC Classics material, and to see the similarities and differences between the TCC Classics and these two major sources of inspiration, the one being mystical and spiritual, and the other direct and pragmatic.

The conclusion looks at TCC as it was, as it is, and as it may become in both the Far East and in the West.

I have tried to keep the book as simple as possible without sacrificing detail. For those unfamiliar with Chinese terms there is a glossary. I have avoided the use of Chinese texts, as this book is aimed at practitioners rather than sinologists; the original classical texts are on my website. Likewise, those who wish to do further reading – and there is much to read – can find an extensive book list there. A common language is shared by Chinese martial arts, Chinese philosophy, Internal Alchemy and meditation. The use of romanization rather than unsatisfactory English language equivalents makes these connections clearer.

It is said that there are four stages in the learning process. The first is unconscious incompetence, where we don't know we don't know how. The second stage is after we have started to learn and to become conscious of our incompetence. Next is the conscious competence stage where we can do it, but only with great concentration. Finally we become unconsciously competent, able to do it without thinking. I hope this offering will aid others on their paths through the stages.

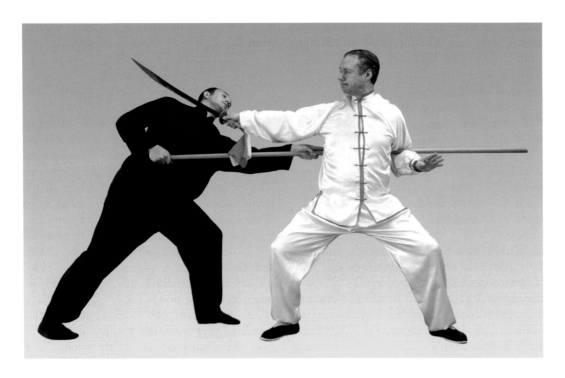

Author demonstrates Sweep across a Thousand Troops.

PART I

BACKGROUND

1   Chinese Martial Arts

Chinese martial arts have existed for well over 3,000 years. Wrestling and swordsmanship both have a long history, as do Chinese Internal Alchemy and breathing methods. These disparate elements, married by Yin Yang theory, became what we now call Tai Chi Chuan.

Most people in the West use the term '*Kung Fu*' to refer to Chinese martial arts. The character for *Kung/Gong* is a combination of the characters for work and strength, and therefore implies 'that which is meritorious'. '*Fu*' is man. Kung Fu refers to skill or workmanship in any field, including that of martial arts. '*Wushu*' is the literal term for martial art in Chinese, but has come to be associated with the gymnastic, acrobatic and dance-like silk-suited performances of modern competition *Wushu*. Other terms used as such include *Chuan/Quan Shu* (fist/ art) and *Kuo/Guo Shu* (national art).

Chinese Kung Fu is often divided into soft/internal and hard/external. The former is often identified with the Taoist enclave of Wudang Mountain, and the latter with the Shaolin Chan Buddhist temples. Internal arts such as TCC have external or Yang elements just as external arts have internal elements.

Many Chinese martial arts came neither from Wudang nor Shaolin, so this division and these associations are not definitive.

Patriot, scholar-philosopher, politician and martial artist, Huang Zong-xi (1610–95) gave the classical definition of external and internal martial arts. In 1669 as part of a tombstone epitaph for his master, Wang Zheng-nan, Huang wrote:

> Shaolin is famous under Heaven for the courage of its boxing, so it aims at attacking others... In the so-called Internal Family (*Nei Jia*), stillness is used to control movement; when the opponent attacks then he is countered. Therefore Shaolin is called External Family (*Wai Jia*).

Huang then traces the internal system to the Taoist, Chang San-feng, though the dates he gives for Chang are obviously wrong. The distinction between 'external' and 'internal' is also referred to in Classic 2, while Classic 5 outlines the quintessential internal martial arts approach to fighting.

TCC, *Ba Gua Zhang* (Eight Trigram Palm) and *XingYi* (Form and Intent Boxing) are the main styles identified as internal, and enjoy

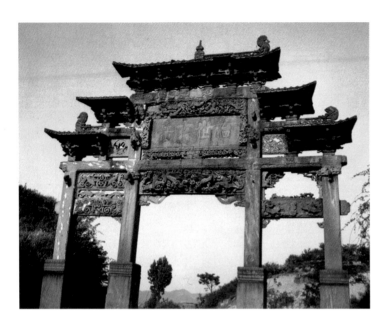

Fig. 1 Old entrance gate to Wudang Mountain.

some similarities in approach (not just martial technique, but also meditative and Internal Alchemy practices), jargon and terminology, and mnemonic Classics. Other reasons given for considering Shaolin to be external, and TCC, *Bagua Zhang* (Eight Trigram Palm) and *XingYi* (Form and Intent) to be internal, is that Shaolin is Buddhist and so foreign. In addition, monks had to go out from family and society, while the other arts are native to China and did not require the practitioner to leave his family and society.

Typically, we can divide the syllabus of a Chinese martial art into various aspects. The most familiar is forms (*Taolu*, or *Tao Chuan/ Quan*), where the adept practises a sequence of choreographed martial movements, which can last anything from some seconds to half an hour or more. Forms can be done vigorously or softly, quickly or slowly, flamboyantly or simply. There are both weapon and hand forms.

San Shou, which can be translated as 'dispersing/scattering the hands' or 'hands which disperse/scatter', comprises all the unarmed fighting techniques of a particular art, whether striking, kicking, throwing, locking or parrying. Be clear: techniques do not come from forms; forms come from techniques. Many TCC techniques are hidden or performed quite differently in forms than in application.

Aspects of *San Shou* include *Shuai Jiao*, which involves throwing, tripping and sweeping; *Qinna*, which means to seize and hold, and is concerned with controlling, locking and restraining an opponent, often to set up a percussive strike; and *Diepu*, making the opponent fall by hitting him, or hitting him when he has fallen.

In the term *Dim Mak* (Cantonese) or *Dian Xue* (Mandarin), *Dim/Dian* means a/to point/ dot, and *Mak/Xue* means a hole/vital point, or to bore a hole. It is often called pressure points; these are attacked by hitting, gripping, tearing or pressing selected points of the body, thus causing internal bleeding, paralysis, unconsciousness and even death. Many people over-complicate all this and bring in acupuncture points, meridians and the time

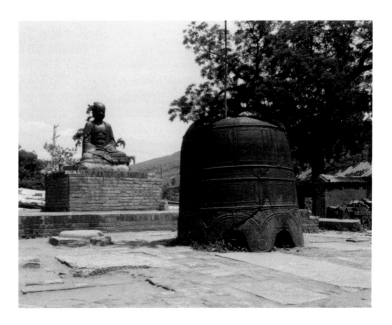

Fig. 2 Ruin of Shaolin Temple in 1984.

of day, but it is mainly about concentrating force precisely on a vein, artery, nerve, joint or vital point such as the philtrum. It is not a secret art; most people just don't have the skill or accuracy to do it effectively.

There are two types of offensive *Dim Mak*: the first involves short or long range striking of an opponent's anatomy; the second involves the sudden or sharp use of force by gripping or twisting. Both methods aim to render the opponent incapable of offering further resistance, or to set up another technique. This gripping and twisting is *Qinna*.

Most Chinese martial arts have methods to control an opponent at close quarters; this is both grabbing and hitting distance. Praying Mantis and *Wing Chun* employ 'sticking hands' training; internal systems and particularly TCC use 'pushing hands' (*Tui Shou*) training. Controlling an opponent at a close distance also sets up an opportunity for *Dim Mak*. Pushing hands trains timing, distance, footwork and in-fighting. Free pushing hands is mainly concerned with unbalancing, but sometimes also with throwing, striking or locking an opponent. There are now competitions in this all over the world. I have been running the British Open Tai Chi Championships since 1989. Competition pushing hands events include both fixed step (competitors keep their feet more or less fixed) and moving step (competitors may move within a set area).

The three classical Chinese martial arts weapons are the spear, the sabre/broadsword and the double-edged straight sword; all three of these are part of the syllabus in most traditional schools of Tai Chi Chuan. There is an old Chinese boxing saying: 'Spear 100 days. Sabre 1,000 days. Sword 10,000 days.' This expresses the degree of difficulty of each. In many weapon forms there are elements of *Qinna*, *Shuai Jiao*, *Tui Shou* and even *Dim Mak*. All these aspects are interrelated.

The most important element in Chinese martial arts is *Kung/Gong* training, or what gives the 'Kung Fu'. There is a well known maxim: 'Learn boxing (*Chuan*), but don't train conditioning (*Kung/Gong*), even till old age it is still empty.' Techniques are not

13

enough; you need to have the power to take and give techniques effectively.

Qigong/Chi Kung is training involving *Qi* – exercises and postures to improve respiration and circulation. In many external systems such as Shaolin, *Qigong/Chi Kung* methods involve deep breathing and dynamic tension. All traditional Chinese martial arts have some type of martial *Kung/Gong* training. There are many excellent non-martial *Nei/Qi Kung/Gong* methods. Many martial *Kung/Gong*, such as Tai Chi Nei Kung (Internal Strength), also contain meditative, health, ritual and Internal Alchemy elements. Tai Chi Nei Kung relies more on total body force and correct posture for strengthening the body, developing martial skill and the ability to give and receive blows. The influence of meditation and Internal Alchemy on TCC practice will be discussed later.

Taoism has deeply influenced oriental martial arts. Japanese martial arts are divided into '*Do*' and '*Jutsu*': *Do* is the same character as the Chinese '*Tao*', meaning way or

ways, while '*Jutsu*' means technique. Ken-do, Ju-do and Aiki-do are supposedly more concerned with martial arts as spiritual development and a way of life, and there is a strong Zen Buddhist influence. Ju Jutsu, Karate Jutsu and other *Jutsu* are supposedly only concerned with combat efficacy and are not martial arts, but pure fighting. Most Ju Jutsu practised today comes from the art taught by the Chinese master, Chen Yuan-bin, to three samurai in Nagasaki in 1638. Ju Jutsu (techniques of softness) is exactly the TCC concept of Yin defeating Yang by using the opponent's own force against him; even *Jutsu* are not immune to Taoist philosophy.

The influence of Taoist theory on the TCC Classics is such that TCC can be very much a 'way' as opposed to the approach found in military manuals such as the *Classic of Boxing*, where, as is supposedly the case with '*Jutsu*', the emphasis is on practicality and there is no spiritual or therapeutic aspect. The *Classic of Boxing* will be discussed in Part III.

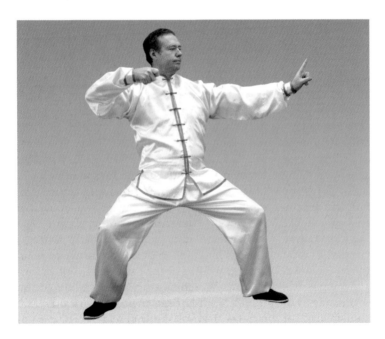

Author demonstrates Taoist Qigong.

2 Chinese Cultural Context

Chinese often refer to the 'Three Teachings' of Confucianism, Buddhism and Taoism. All have philosophical and ritualistic or religious elements. Other important schools of philosophy include the eponymous Legalists, who regulated every action with laws and punishments; the Mohists, who professed universal love and aimed to do only what was practical; and the Dialecticians who heavily influenced the cryptic *Koans* of Chan Buddhism. However, the Three Teachings were, and are, pre-eminent in their influence: these schools influenced one another, and many literati moved easily from one to another.

Confucius wished to educate the ruler, and through him the people, about regulating correct conduct in society and paying attention to the rites to be followed. His doctrines are still used today in Chinese, Japanese and Korean society, though often in a perverse way. It is an irony of history that Confucius was a failure in his professional life; he was an 'Inner Sage', who, though unknown in his life, lived on through his teachings. I once visited his home town of Qufu in Shandong where successive emperors erected mansions and shrines to honour him, and where for centuries his descendants lived, who were given imperial positions in honour of the unsuccessful sage. They became custodians, yet prisoners of his memory. The same is true today of many martial arts schools.

Buddhism is concerned with achieving enlightenment and, through it, freedom from the wheel of reincarnation. Taoism can be divided into religious and practical. Religious Taoism involves incantations, exorcisms and a strong occult element; practical Taoism is concerned with humanity being in harmony with heaven above and earth below.

The stereotypical Confucian scholar was solemn and pompous, prosaic and dull; moralistic, but possessing common sense; a conscientious bureaucrat and family man. The Taoist wanderer or recluse was a carefree spirit, escaping from respectability and conventional duties, a person of wit and paradox, mystical and poetic. The latter stereotype was often found in the same scholar gentleman, away from the demands of society and intoxicated by wine or nature.

My master's uncle, Cheng Wing-kwong, was fascinated by *Qigong* as well as TCC, and learned Immortal Family Eight Pieces of Brocade, which includes sexual exercises, from a wandering Taoist. Cheng told the Taoist that he, too, wanted to be a Taoist. The man then said him, 'Come with me.' Cheng replied, 'Where are we going? What about my family and my business?' – and was told that he had already failed in his ambition.

Stories tell of how in former times students were tested by the master. The diet and the physical regimen were often tough, and in my visits to martial arts schools in China, it has been evident that there is an element of brutality in the treatment of students. The Chinese call the endurance of such hardship 'eating bitterness' and believe it helps to build the character: this is not to

15

say that sentient pleasures are forbidden, but the primary sentient pleasure is good health, hence the Taoist emphasis on both Internal and External Alchemy.

The Three Teachings are not entirely separate entities. The *Book of Changes* (*I Ching*/*Yi Jing*) is widely seen as Taoist because it deals with the duality of Yin and Yang – yet Confucius was devoted to its study, and there was a ritual method of consulting it. Confucianism gave a code of conduct to Buddhist and Taoist hierarchies, including martial arts communities. In the interplay between Buddhism and Taoism, Chan Buddhism and the Complete Reality School of Taoism borrowed heavily from one another. In 1984 I saw Tai Chi symbols at the Chan Buddhist Shaolin Temple, and a Buddhist swastika carved on an incense burner at a Taoist temple on Wudang Mountain.

Society is run by codes: religious, moral and legal. My teacher used the ancient practice of *Bai Shi* (the ritual initiation of disciples) in his school, as I continue to do. The paradox is that while the code of *Bai Shi* emphasizes that TCC comes from Taoism, its emphasis on respect for teachers and senior members of the school, and on correct behaviour, is straight from Confucianism, as is the ritual ceremony of initiation. Similar, more complex codes and rituals are found in many Taoist sects. Many of the 'rules' on how to do TCC found in the TCC Classics, and even the titles of a couple of the TCC Classics, come from Chinese philosophy.

A martial form (choreographed sequence) is image, while combat application of the form's specific and recognizable techniques is reality; but forms are also aesthetic manifestations of *Kung Fu* – strength or skill acquired by meritorious effort. Many practitioners fail to understand that form techniques are rarely applied exactly as they appear in said form. Often there are permitted variations, of different degrees of

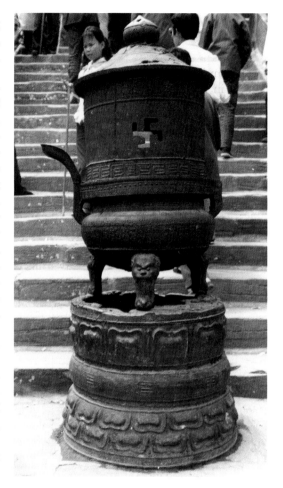

Fig. 3 Incense burner with swastika on Wudang Mountain.

technical and gymnastic difficulty. We have pictures of famous teachers such as Yang Cheng-fu showing ridiculous applications of techniques, which exactly mirror the form movements. These pictures are often taken at face value and people wonder why the applications don't work. They are in prisons and museums of their own construction.

TCC brother Ian Cameron once explained that he was trying to pare down technique, to aim for the simplicity of a Zen painting (he is an ordained Zen Buddhist priest).

The idea in painting is not to paint an exact copy of the subject but to convey its essence, not necessarily by simplification – except at the beginning – but by subtlety. Many techniques in my own lineage are applied with the reverse movements to those in the form, which is one of the reasons why we also practise reverse form.

It is a Taoist truism that if there were no laws there would be no criminals. How then to deal with what is unacceptable? In competition fighting, I usually followed the rules. In 1980, when fighting an old opponent from *Chikechuan* (a blend of Choy Li Fat and Thai boxing) in Kuala Lumpur, I deliberately kicked him in the groin. He had done the same thing to me at the beginning of the first round, but despite my protests, the referee did nothing. Four years previously in Singapore, I was hurt after my first fight, so I deliberately punched my next Shaolin opponent in the face with a twisting action aimed at cutting him. The fight was stopped, his face cut above and below both eyes. Which action was the worse? Tricky things, rules.

There is a Taoist story of a man who wishes to cross a ditch during a deluge: using a fallen stele of the local god to bridge the divide, he walks over to the other side. Another man arrives and finding the fallen stele covered with muddy footprints, cleans it and reverently restores it to its rightful place. In the Taoist pantheon another god asks the local god, 'And so you will punish the first man and reward the second one?' The local god replies, 'I can do nothing to the first man because he does not believe in me. I will punish the second one.'

Belief in codes, rules and ways is a dangerous thing, almost as dangerous as telling the truth.

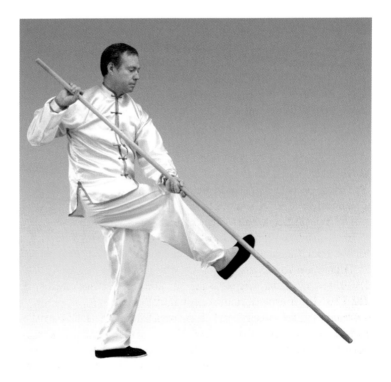

Author demonstrates
Celestial Horse walks
the Skies.

17

3 Philosophical Origins of Tai Chi Chuan Theory

The term 'Tai Chi Chuan' suggests a martial art (*Chuan* means 'fist' and, by extension, a way of fighting) based on the way of harmonious interaction of Yin and Yang. Many books stress the link between TCC and Taoist philosophy and practice; however, the genesis of TCC is not from Taoism alone, but also from strands of Confucian, Dialectic and Neo-Confucian thought. The original *Book of Changes* (*I Ching/Yi Jing*) as a text for divination dates to some time between the eleventh and fifteenth centuries BC; appendices of a more philosophical nature were added later. The *Book of Changes* is not strictly a Taoist text, but is developed from divination texts into a Confucian classic. The first known reference to Tai Chi in Chinese literature is in Appendix III of the *Book of Changes*, which dates from around the second century BC. It states:

> The *I* (Book of Changes) has *Tai Chi* (the Great Ultimate),
> It gives birth to the Two Principles (*ie* Yin and Yang).
> The Two Principles give birth to the Four Emblems;
> The Four Emblems give birth to the Eight Trigrams.

Tai Chi is a Chinese philosophical concept representing the origin of Heaven and Earth and all matter in the world. The character 'Tai' means 'supreme', while 'Chi' has the meaning of 'ultimate' or 'pole', as in ridge pole or North Pole; it is also a reference to the pole star of Ursa Major, a constellation of great significance to the Chinese.

For many Chinese, the genesis of the universe is to be found in the interaction between the two complementary forces within Tai Chi: Yin and Yang. Yin is perceived as female/soft/negative, Yang as male/hard/positive. They are known as '*Liang Yi*', or Two Principles. In the Tai Chi motif shown in Fig. 4, the white half on the left side represents Yang, while the black half on the right side represents Yin. The black spot on the white half is the Yin in the Yang; the white spot on the black half is the Yang in the Yin.

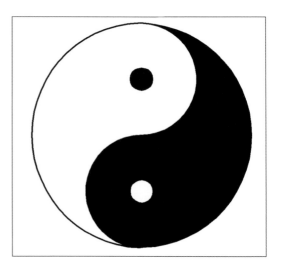

Fig. 4 Tai Chi Motif.

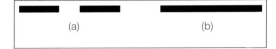

Fig. 5 (a) Yin line. (b) Yang line.

A single Yin line with a single Yang line is also referred to as the Two Principles. The Yin line represents the black half of the Tai Chi motif, whereas the Yang line represents the white half.

The Two Principles interact to produce change and give rise to *Si Xiang*, the Four Emblems, each represented by two lines. These Four Emblems are responsible for the formation of the universe, and can be classified as Old Yin, Young Yang, Young Yin and Old Yang.

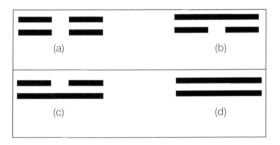

Fig. 6 (a) Old Yin. (b) Young Yang. (c) Young Yin. (d) Old Yang.

The interaction of Yin and Yang also causes the formation from the Four Emblems of eight more entities that affect the growth of plants, the birth of animals, and even the evolution of the human race. These entities are known as the Eight Trigrams (*Ba Gua*) and are shown in Fig. 7.

The completion of the *Book of Changes* (*I Ching/Yi Jing*) was also based on the theory of Tai Chi. The process by which, in a logical sequence, the sixty-four hexagrams of the *Book of Changes* were derived from the Tai Chi motif and the Eight Trigrams is reproduced in Fig. 8; it is a sequence that can be continued *ad infinitum*. Taoists believed that in this way all matter could be traced back to the Tai Chi motif.

Yin and Yang are complementary opposites and are the two factors that combine to form Tai Chi. If we divide the abstract concept of Tai Chi into Yin and Yang, we can use it to examine the universe and all the matter in it. Yin signifies softness, stillness, interior, Earth, darkness, night, the female principle and negative polarity; Yang signifies hardness, motion, exterior, Heaven, light, day, the male principle and positive polarity.

In a favourable environment Yin and Yang will interact and develop; in an unfavourable

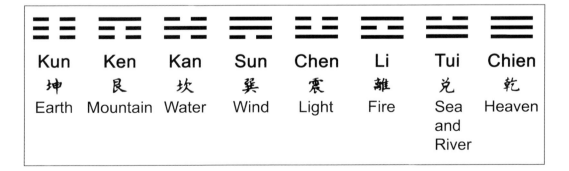

Fig. 7 The Eight Trigrams.

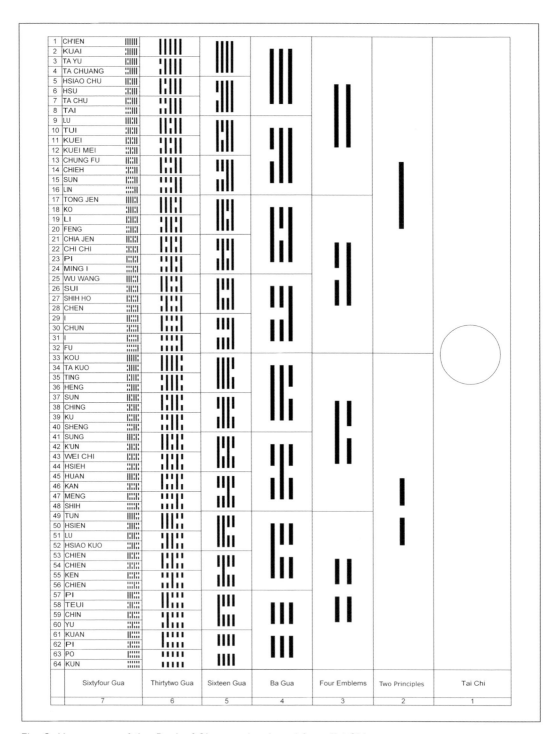

	Sixtyfour Gua	Thirtytwo Gua	Sixteen Gua	Ba Gua	Four Emblems	Two Principles	Tai Chi
1 CH'IEN							
2 KUAI							
3 TA YU							
4 TA CHUANG							
5 HSIAO CHU							
6 HSU							
7 TA CHU							
8 TAI							
9 LU							
10 TUI							
11 KUEI							
12 KUEI MEI							
13 CHUNG FU							
14 CHIEH							
15 SUN							
16 LIN							
17 TONG JEN							
18 KO							
19 LI							
20 FENG							
21 CHIA JEN							
22 CHI CHI							
23 PI							
24 MING I							
25 WU WANG							
26 SUI							
27 SHIH HO							
28 CHEN							
29 I							
30 CHUN							
31 I							
32 FU							
33 KOU							
34 TA KUO							
35 TING							
36 HENG							
37 SUN							
38 CHING							
39 KU							
40 SHENG							
41 SUNG							
42 K'UN							
43 WEI CHI							
44 HSIEH							
45 HUAN							
46 KAN							
47 MENG							
48 SHIH							
49 TUN							
50 HSIEN							
51 LU							
52 HSIAO KUO							
53 CHIEN							
54 CHIEN							
55 KEN							
56 CHIEN							
57 PI							
58 TEUI							
59 CHIN							
60 YU							
61 KUAN							
62 PI							
63 PO							
64 KUN							
	7	6	5	4	3	2	1

Fig. 8 Hexagrams of the *Book of Changes* developed from Tai Chi.

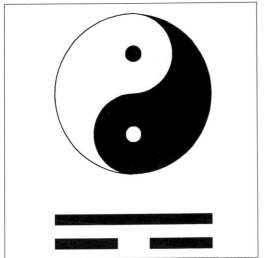

Fig. 9 Young Yang.

Fig. 10 Old Yang.

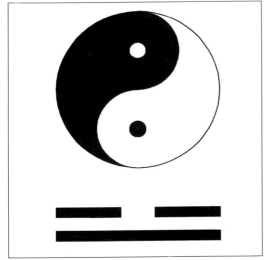

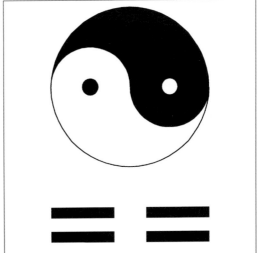

Fig. 11 Young Yin.

Fig. 12 Old Yin.

environment they will repel one another and destroy all matter. Yin and Yang counteract and yet interact. When in any one situation their interaction reaches a conclusion, the natural phenomena in that situation will follow a pattern of variation in constant repetition, as is shown by the diagrams in Figs

9–12. These diagrams, in representing the changes of Yin and Yang, are called the Four Emblems.

Figure 9 has Yang ascending while Yin is descending. Yang here represents spring, brightness and the sun; in terms of time, it is the morning of the day. This is why this

MONTH	SEASON	TIME	TAI CHI MOTIF	HEXAGRAM
1	Early Spring	6 am		TAI
2	Mid Spring	8 am		TA CHUANG
3	Late Spring	10 am		KUAI
4	Early Summer	12 am		CHIEN
5	Mid Summer	2 pm		KOU
6	Late Summer	4 pm		TUN
7	Early Autumn	6 pm		PI
8	Mid Autumn	8 pm		KUAN
9	Late Autumn	10 pm		PO
10	Early Winter	12 pm		KUN
11	Mid Winter	2 am		FU
12	Late Winter	4 am		LIN

Fig. 13 The waxing and waning of Yin and Yang on the Chinese calendar.

propitious motif is normally adopted by Tai Chi Chuan schools.

Figure 10 has Yang on top while Yin is underneath. This is Yang at its strongest point, where it completely dominates Yin. This means the sun is at its zenith and the time is noon; it is now summer time.

Figure 11 has Yang descending while Yin is ascending. Yin represents the moon and darkness, so it is now dusk; the brightness of the sun is on the wane, the leaves are falling and autumn has come.

Figure 12 has Yang at its nadir while Yin has reached its zenith. Yin has followed Yang as night follows day. The time is now midnight. Old Yin will be followed by Young Yang. Winter is now with us.

Figures 9–12 show the Tai Chi symbol rotating clockwise in a generative cycle. When the symbol rotates anticlockwise, it represents a destructive cycle. These cycles are explained later, in the commentary to Classic 1, when discussing Five Elements theory.

Chinese New Year begins at the end of January or beginning of February, and is seen as the beginning of spring. Spring and summer are times of growth and activity and so represent Yang. Autumn and winter are periods of decline and passivity and so represent Yin. The changes of Yin and Yang during the Chinese lunar year can be shown using the hexagrams of the *Book of Changes* and the Tai Chi motif. The changes of the Tai Chi motif are shown in two ways in Fig. 13, the left central column representing the inevitable and continuous nature of the complementary changes of Yin and Yang.

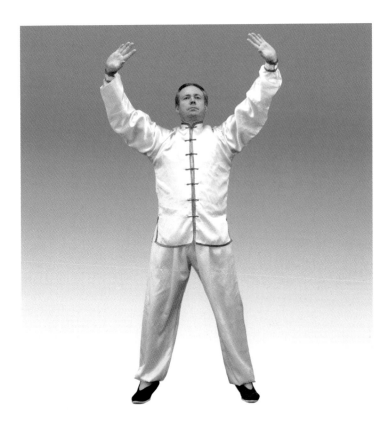

Author demonstrates Support the Sky from Taoist Qigong.

4 The Inner Way and Ways

Normally '*Tao*' is translated as 'The Way'. Taoists are followers of The Way, but there are many ways and many types of Taoism, and not every way is equally suitable and efficacious for everybody. Inner ways include *Qigong*, Internal Alchemy, meditation and prayer. It is often difficult to see where the divide between these practices occurs. For *Qigong* alone there are hundreds of systems

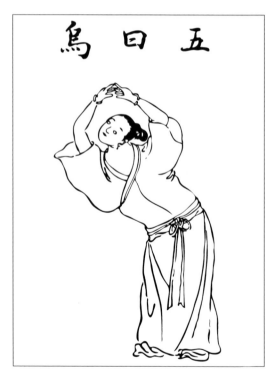

Fig. 14 Bird exercise from Five Animal Frolic.

incorporating martial, ritualistic, religious, Internal Alchemy, shamanistic, therapeutic and meditative elements. One of the earliest methods was the Five Animal Frolic, attributed to the famous physician Hua Tuo (third century BC).

The relationship between TCC and Taoism is in philosophical, alchemical, meditative and martial practices, and not religious practices such as exorcism or prayer. On Wudang Mountain there was even a prison for Taoist priests and others who broke the regulations set by the abbots and by imperial decree. When I visited in 2004, it had been turned into a martial arts school.

In meditative and Internal Alchemy practice there are different levels. In Tai Chi Nei Kung there are three levels for each exercise: for beginners, for adepts and for masters.

Tai Chi Chuan and Chinese Alchemy

External Alchemy (*Wai Dan*) uses drugs, medicines and plants to produce effects on the body or mind, and is an important part of Chinese medicine and Taoist practice. It was a part of shamanic rituals. Before fighting in Chinese full contact in South East Asia, I ate ginseng and afterwards took papaya to balance out the Yang quality of the ginseng. In Singapore in 1976 I was offered anabolic steroids by my teacher and refused to take them, but I did eat bear gall bladder and had moxibustion treatment after getting

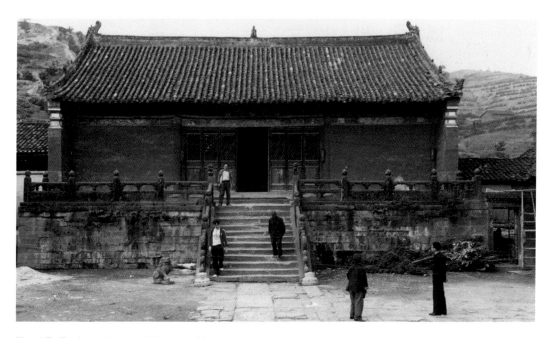

Fig. 15 Taoist prison on Wudang Mountain.

badly beaten up in my first fight – which I won.

A practice common to many types of Taoism, and important in TCC, is that of *Nei Dan*, or Internal Alchemy. There are references as far back as Chuang Tzu (c. fifth century BC) to breathing exercises, and unverifiable claims that some Internal Alchemy exercises had an even greater antiquity. The theme of Internal Alchemy runs through all but the last of the TCC Classics – which is not surprising, as it is entitled the Fighter's Song.

Another name for Internal Alchemy is *Dao Yin* (Leading and Conducting (energy)). In 1973 in a Han tomb dated to 168BC at Ma Wang Dui, Hunan, a chart was found illustrating a variety of *Dao Yin* exercises; some bore a resemblance to TCC techniques, such as Seven Stars and Single Whip. The main distinction between Internal Alchemy and meditation is that the former is more concerned with energy circulation and transformation, while the latter is more concerned with developing a calm state of mind. Both are *Qigong* as both involve respiration and circulation training.

In Internal Alchemy, the Three Treasures of *Qi*, *Jing* and *Shen* are stimulated by thought, exercise and breath. *Qi* vitalizes the body, while *Jing* in the form of semen, saliva and bodily secretions irrigates it. *Shen* is developed by the Yin Yang method of shutting out the exterior world of the senses and the interior world of thought and emotions, while opening ourselves to the spiritual world of the infinite.

Some practitioners try to direct *Qi* to acupoints or to the lower *Dantian* (Cinnabar Field), just below the navel (*Dan* in *Dantian* is the same character as in *Nei Dan* and *Wai Dan* and so a reference to alchemy). Others visualize converting *Qi* to *Jing* to *Shen* as the energy travels along microcosmic or macrocosmic orbits. Yet others practise *Zhan Zhuang*, meaning standing meditation/ Pile-Stance training, a practice sometimes

25

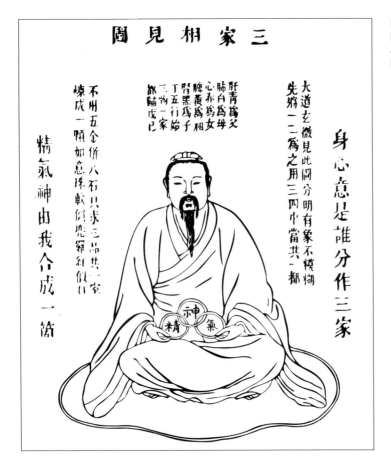

三家相見圖

精氣神由我合成一箇

不卅五全併八石以求三品共一室 憭成一順如意珠轉似兜羅紅似

斂歛三物丁心脾腎肺肝
戊一五白黃黑白青
己家始行為為為為
子祖女母父

大道玄微見此圖分明有象不模糊
失將一二為之用三四中當共一都

身心意是誰分作三家

神
精 氣

Fig. 16 Taoist adept holding, from left, *Jing*, *Shen* and *Qi*. Note the links between them.

referred to as 'tree-hugging'. This practice may well have come from *Xing Yi* (Form and Intent) boxing or one of its offshoots.

In Internal Alchemy, males and females are sometimes advised to practise certain exercises differently, and in some cases they practise different exercises entirely. In certain types of TCC training males are expected to abstain from sex for 100 days; females are not, because their supply of *Jing* is considered to be limitless, although practice can affect, and be affected by, the menstrual cycle.

In developing detachment, some schools of Taoism focus on a specific area or point of the body, such as a cavity or the *Dantian*. In trying to move energy around the body, some schools visualize and use metaphors such as the 'Sea of *Qi*' in the lower *Dantian*; 'Needle at Sea Bottom' is a reference to a groin strike to this point.

TCC is identified with abdominal breathing. Internal Alchemy methods such as 'Emptying the Mind and Filling the Belly' suppress emotions and fill the lower *Dan Tian* with energy by controlling the breath and drawing essences from sexual partners and celestial bodies. The TCC Classics specifically tell us to let the *Qi* sink to the *Dan Tian*. They also advise that the *Shen* be internally hoarded, and that we use a partner's or opponent's force against him; sexual manuals

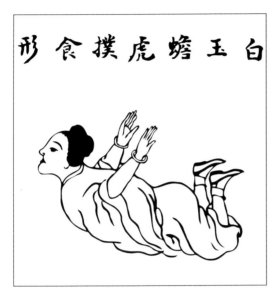

形食撲虎蟾玉白

Fig. 17 Female adept practising Taoist Internal Alchemy cultivation.

advised similar tactics when trying to satisfy wives and concubines.

In 'Uniting Intention and Breath' at an advanced level, the duality between the adept and the universal energy of the Tao is dissolved, so there is no separation of external and internal, and there is only one breath, the breath of Tao, the source of life. This expresses the meaning of 'Tai Chi in Unity' at the end of TCC forms. The whole body is one breath as opposed to breathing only with the nostrils, lungs, and so on. In TCC practice correct breathing does not normally involve conscious thought, and the concentration is not on the breath, but on relaxation and correct posture. The breathing pattern is dictated by the speed and the nature of the techniques or postures.

The TCC Classics talk of *Qi* entering the bones. Medical research shows that bone mass density can be maintained amongst older people by regular exercise, making the bones softer and less brittle. In the same way, 'Gathering and Circulating the Light of the Spirit', an advanced Internal Alchemy of the Complete Reality School, seeks to strengthen and soften the bones to increase and transform *Qi*, *Jing* and *Shen*.

Training is often demanding. 'Returning to Earlier Heaven' as practised by the Way of Earlier Heaven Sect involves specific rigorous postures; equal importance is placed on cultivating body and mind. Hand positions include sitting with the hands on the knees and holding them together to form a Tai Chi symbol, or supporting the body on the knuckles while in a full lotus.

In Tai Chi Nei Kung meditation we also sit sometimes with the hands on the knees and hold the cupped hands together, as if holding a Tai Chi symbol or a lotus. Doing handstands on the knuckles is a TCC conditioning practice to develop solid punching. This mix of therapeutic and martial elements, as well as meditative and alchemical ones, makes TCC a very complex art.

Internal Alchemy can involve meditation, but also aims to strengthen the skeletal system and regulate the internal physiology, as opposed to 'pure' meditation. As with Tai Chi Nei Kung, it is usually only taught after a disciple has undergone ritual initiation with a master, and then under constant supervision; such practices can be dangerous if done incorrectly.

The phrase 'Walk Fire Enter Demon' refers to practising incorrectly and then suffering side effects. Internal Alchemy sometimes attempts to override the autonomic nervous system, and a malfunction can result in paranoia, spontaneous ejaculation and obsessive-compulsive behaviour. I knew a number of such cases while living in Hong Kong, and have seen the same in the West. It is important to seek out a suitably qualified person before undertaking such training, and to stop and seek advice if problems are encountered.

In 1852, when Yang Lu-chan went to the Qing Imperial Court in Beijing, there was considerable interest in Internal Alchemy amongst the cultural élite. We may well ponder on what exactly Yang was teaching the Emperor's brother and other members of the royal household, compared with the martial material he was teaching to his Imperial Guard students. This is not idle speculation.

In 1980 as part of a book entitled *Wu Family Tai Chi Chuan*, Wu Gung-zao included '*Tai Chi Fa Shuo*', 'An Explanation of Tai Chi Methods'. This purported to be a photocopy of a handwritten collection of forty short texts that his father, Wu Jian-quan, copied from originals passed from Yang Ban-hou to his grandfather, Wu Quan-you. The first page of the photocopy is dated 1948. Wu Jian Quan died in 1942.

Most of the texts dealt with TCC theory and martial methods, but the last three are supposed to come from TCC patriarch, Chang San-feng, and contain many Internal Alchemy references including sexual ones, which seem to advocate congress with male and female prepubescent virgins. Prior to Wu Gung-zao's book, the Yang family had only published twenty-four of the texts. One wonders where the material came from originally, and if the famous TCC families are really practising these methods, which by publication they seem to endorse.

Tai Chi Chuan and Taoist Meditation

Zen ('*Chan*' in Chinese) meditation is a well known aspect of Japanese culture, especially favoured by the Samurai warrior class, and used to train detachment and spontaneity. Less is known of the connections between TCC and Taoist meditation.

Meditation is part of the *Yang Sheng* (Nourishing of Life) practice referred to by Taoist philosopher, Chuang Tzu, in the fifth century BC. The master–disciple relationship in Chinese culture is often referred to as one of father and son, because metaphorically, the master gives birth to (*Sheng*) and nourishes (*Yang*) the disciple. Sickness arises from a lack, an excess or blockage of *Jing* or *Qi*, so many Taoists sought purification and tranquillity through ritual washing, fasting and withdrawal to the mountainous domain of the gods from an impure world, there to meditate.

Taoists see meditation as going from movement to stillness and from stillness to movement. Likewise in TCC hand form, we go from briefly holding the *Wu Chi* (No Ultimate) position (also known as Tai Chi at Rest) to holding briefly the Ready/ Tai Chi position, and then commence the form. We finish the form by going from Tai Chi in Unity back to *Wu Chi* (also known as Completion Style). Famous master Sun Lu-tang (1861–1932) wrote that before practising internal martial arts, in the state of *Wu Chi*, there was no thought, no intent, no form and so no shape. These stylized and seemingly unimportant form transitions are triggers that induce the focus and concentration needed to do the form properly, and to unwind after the journey is complete.

Likewise there are ritual opening and closing sequences in Tai Chi Nei Kung. In addition after each exercise, we return to the 'Embracing the One' (*Bao Yi*) position before commencing the next exercise. 'Embracing the One' is a direct quotation from Lao Tzu's *Tao Te Ching* (Classic of the Way and Virtue) and is the exact name of a static posture of Tai Chi Nei Kung, which might be held initially for a few minutes and later for up to half an hour with the eyes shut. The term also appears in a number of texts from the Complete Reality School of Taoism. Interestingly, TCC founder, Chang San-feng, was a member of the Complete Reality School.

The Highest Purity sect practises 'Embracing the One' by visualizing manifestations of the Tao, such as Lao Tzu, to keep the deity/

spirit within oneself. When Embracing the One, the adept achieves oneness by dissolving the duality of self and the world and by filling the mind and body so that no thoughts, emotions or sensations can arise. Once stillness is attained, one can attain immortality, where all things are seen as one. This method emphasizes the stillness of body and mind during practice because movement destroys the experience of oneness. This physically demanding method requires a strong spine because adepts might hold one position for long periods.

Oneness is highly important in Taoist meditation. In 'Holding/Keeping the One' (*Shou Yi*), or 'Acquiring the One' (*De Yi*), 'One' is the Taoist trinity of Heaven, Earth and Humanity united harmoniously as the Tao. TCC itself is a method to 'Hold/Keep the Way' (*Shou Tao*). With the concept of 'Heaven, Earth, Humanity harmonize as One' (*Tian Di Ren He Yi*), we as humanity composed of Yin and Yang are rooted (by our feet) to the Supreme Yin of Earth, and with *Shen* rising to the head-top, aspire to the Supreme Yang of Heaven. This process is explained in the TCC Classics.

'*Nei Guan*' (Internal Observation) dates from the Tang dynasty (AD618–906). Practitioners try to observe (*Guan*) and be aware of the existence and effects of thoughts and emotions, then learn to stop them arising so that the mind is clear. It is often practised in a lotus position, though it is sometimes done sitting, standing or walking. The walking aspect has a parallel in TCC form practice and the *Bagua Zhang* (Eight Trigram Palm) method of walking the circle.

The term '*Guan*' occurs again in '*Ding Guan*' (Fixed/Tranquil Observation). *Ding* refers to a Yin or Earth-like stability of fixed concentration, which combines with a Yang or Heaven-inspired intuitive wisdom produced by *Guan*. In the TCC Classics, *Ding* appears in the term *Zhong Ding* (Central Stability/Equilibrium), which is identified with the element Earth. Just as the other elements are found in or on the earth, so going forwards or back, left or right, all comes from *Zhong Ding*. Thus movement proceeds from, and back to, stillness.

Meditation is also called 'Storing/Preserving Thoughts' (*Cun Si*), and 'Thinking on Preservation' (*Xiang Cun*). These terms suggest the type of visualization or focusing on words or mantras common to both Tai Chi Nei Kung practice, and to certain types of Taoist and Chan meditation.

A common term is 'Repair/Cultivate the Mind' (*Xiu Xin*). Li Guang-xuan, writing in the Sung period on Internal Alchemy, said that you shouldn't worry about becoming immortal, but should just try to perfect yourself by practising the techniques, and you would be sure to attain truth. Martial arts are similar, in that repetitions refine the technique so it becomes second nature – what you practise most is what you are most likely to do when under pressure.

A final term is '*Zuo Wang*'. *Zuo* means to sit, while *Wang* is to forget or to escape the mind. *Zuo Wang* is closer to the common conception of seated meditation. In Tai Chi Nei Kung training we don't consciously empty the mind, but rather let it wander freely, or focus it by chanting the TCC Classics.

Tai Chi Chuan Practice: Inner Ways and the Senses

Meditation is a way of cultivating health and longevity, of clearing the mind to attain the highest level of spiritual development: union with the Tao. There is a closing of the exterior world of the senses and of the interior world of emotion and thought connected to it, with a simultaneous opening to the universe and the spiritual world.

Meditation can be done privately or in groups, silently or with chanting, and often has spiritual or religious aspects. TCC embraces all these aspects to a greater or lesser degree. Some say that TCC is 'moving meditation', but TCC can be static as well as moving. Furthermore the TCC Classics are mnemonic – that is, designed to be chanted: they express their author's reflections and are guides to others in contemplation of how better to perform TCC. My teacher learned to chant them during Tai Chi Nei Kung practice as a kind of private devotion.

TCC trains the body in movement and also in stillness through practising postures, exercises, forms and drills. This focuses the mind and develops intent. Without focus, techniques are empty gestures. Coordination of the externality of the movements with the internal (breath and intent) develops and controls the Three Treasures – *Qi*, *Jing* and *Shen* – or in Western terms, respiration and circulation, vitality and spirit. The ultimate Taoist and TCC goal is to be empty – that is, free of ego and delusion – so that one can merge with the Tao and attain the state of No Mind (*Wu Xin*).

Sometimes meditation is practised as an introduction to more arduous training, such as certain Internal Alchemy methods; more often it is practised in its own right as an aid to concentration and spiritual development. Sometimes it is practised with the eyes closed, sometimes not.

After training in the theory and practice it becomes possible to pay attention to posture, actions and breathing, whether walking, sitting, standing or reclining; effectively you can practise anytime. The ideal minimum is once a day. I usually practise TCC form in the morning to prepare me for the day ahead, while I prefer to practise TCC meditation late at night because it helps me to sleep.

Sleep can be a real problem. Many years ago a new student told me that he worked irregular hours and needed expensive acupuncture treatment every couple of weeks to help him sleep. I taught him only the first four Yin exercises of Tai Chi Nei Kung, and he had no further problems. Shift workers, including police officers I've taught, have reported similar benefits from these exercises.

It is a paradox that the idea of abstaining from all thought is itself a thought. This is referred to in Chapter 11 of the *Book of the Prince of Huai Nan* (*Huainanzi*, second century BC), which says that those who seek to be emptied cannot be emptied, while those who do not seek it, achieve it spontaneously. In 'Inner Observation', if the eyes are closed they look inwards; likewise the hearing is turned inwards, making it easier to ignore distracting sounds.

Some beginners believe that before they started meditating, thoughts were few and became numerous after taking up meditation. In reality they are more aware of thoughts the more they meditate. Through practice, thoughts eventually decrease. Positive results and health benefits can come from regular meditation, but it is necessary to concentrate on the practice and not try to force it. Success in meditation (as in religion and martial arts) depends upon faith and practice.

TCC breathing is deep on inhalation, and long on exhalation. It should be slow, continuous and almost imperceptible. Taoist sitting meditation and Tai Chi Nei Kung are often preceded by breathing and stretching exercises. With abdominal respiration the lungs expand more than usual, thus taking in more oxygen, which makes the circulation and purification of blood more effective. A higher percentage of carbon dioxide is breathed out or methane gas emitted, and this enhances the development of our Three Treasures of *Qi*, *Jing* and *Shen*.

Some say the longer the meditation the better, and suggest a minimum of thirty minutes. I have practised Tai Chi Nei Kung for between fifteen minutes to three and a half hours most days since 1976, but I rarely practise sitting meditation for more than ten minutes. I believe that long periods of sitting meditation can lead to drowsiness and lassitude, and can damage the knees by cutting off the circulation.

Meditation can help develop kinaesthesis: a kind of sixth sense or feeling of where you are in relation to your body and to external people and objects, whether you or they are static or moving. To test this ability, close the eyes and try to touch the nose with the index finger. Alternatively, time yourself standing on one foot with the eyes open, and do the same thing with the eyes shut. In martial arts we use kinaesthetic ability when we instantaneously judge our timing, distance and position in relation to a stimulus such as an attack.

Ting, or listening, is an interesting term used in TCC to refer to the situation in pushing hands or *San Shou* when we are in physical contact with the opponent and thus able to 'listen to' (feel) his actions and reactions in order to influence or respond to them.

In a truly kinaesthetic process, we can use the regular senses as well as the sixth sense. The eyes see the opponent, the heart or emotions sense him, and the ears hear him (his breath at least). These faculties, combined with the sense of touch (perhaps we can smell him as well, though we don't want to taste him), produce a heightened state of awareness. This is what we mean by listening in a TCC sense.

We can sharpen this 'listening' by closing the eyes during *Tui Shou*, because the primary sense on which we are relying at close quarters is touch rather than sight. This is meditation in action. The eyes are normally closed in five Tai Chi Nei Kung techniques, and I practise form with the eyes closed to develop balance and sensitivity (this practice is common in other martial arts such as karate). In practising with the eyes closed, we have to feel our foot positions on the floor

and orientate ourselves according to any ambient sounds or vibrations, while visualizing the techniques as we do them.

The Chinese habitually practise martial arts and *Qigong* outdoors and wearing shoes, but if we are practising a static form of meditation, we are more prone to be disturbed by the wind, sun and other elements, and by birds and animals. That is why many adepts practised in mountain caves, as is said about Chang San-feng on Wudang Mountain and in Baoji, and Bodhidharma on Songshan. Then, too, because caves were used by wild animals, they were seen as places with very powerful *Qi*.

In the year 2000, on Wudang Mountain, I met a bedridden Taoist nun, Li Cheng Yu, then supposed to be 113 years old. I asked if she had ever practised Tai Chi Chuan. She replied that she had come to the mountain as a young girl, and had at that time practised *Wen* (Cultural) TCC as a daily form of meditative and therapeutic Taoist practice, rather than as a martial art. This holistic approach is rarely found nowadays: people practise without any idea of what they are doing, and have little or no idea about Internal Alchemy, so any meditative aspect is at best superficial.

In the mid-1970s, when walking in the hills around Hong Kong with my master, we often came upon open areas clearly being used for martial arts or *Qigong* practice. Outdoor early morning practice is still common because that is when trees and plants give out oxygen; there are fewer people around at that time; and it readies the practitioner for the day ahead. The summer months are hot and humid, so it is unpleasant to practise during the day. When practising TCC outdoors in the morning, it is best to start off facing west, so the sun is in the face for a minimal amount of time.

Meditation in Chinese society is linked with religious communities. Temples and monasteries are often located in remote

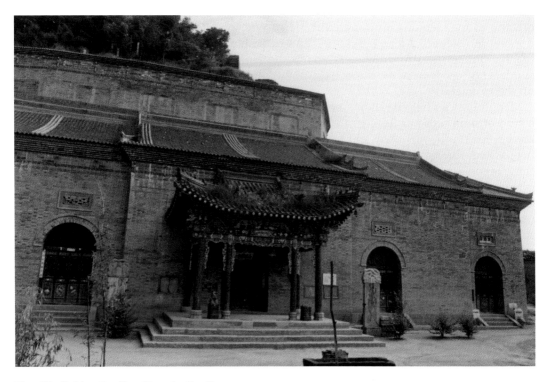

Fig. 18 Golden Pavilion Temple, Baoji.

areas, and were specifically designed for meditation and contemplation. Some, like the Taoist White Cloud Temple in Beijing, are huge, containing many buildings and courtyards. Although situated in the heart of the city, this temple feels a secluded and tranquil place and, not surprisingly, has long been associated with meditation and TCC. Meditation is practised in individual cells or in communal meditation halls. Communal meals, work and other activities with like-minded individuals make it easier to meditate in an enclosed and disciplined community isolated from the temptations of the world of the flesh outside.

For sitting meditation, Taoists often use cushions, but a bed is also suitable. It is not necessary to go into a lotus position; just sitting on the edge of a chair or bed with ankles crossed and knees facing out to open

up the crotch is also fine. When static, the back is normally straight and erect so the spinal column is correctly aligned and the lungs can expand. After meditation the eyes should be opened slowly and the limbs massaged or flexed to relax them.

The hands are often placed palms down on the knees, or one on the other, palms up, close to the belly with the thumbs interlocked. The head and neck should be erect and facing ahead. The eyes are often lightly shut so as to avoid distractions, or are focused on something, while the mouth is closed with the tongue touching the palate, to make a bridge along which *Qi* moves from the nose to the throat, or vice versa. As with TCC practice, we normally breathe in and out through the nose.

A successor of Hua Tuo, the noted alchemist Ko Hung (fourth to fifth century AD),

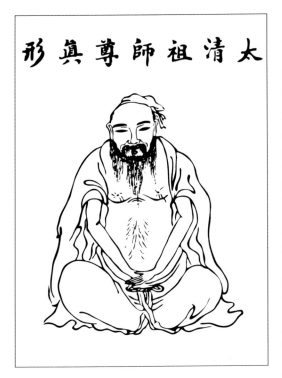

太清祖師尊真形

Fig. 19 Sitting meditation.

in his *Baobuzi* (*Master who Embraces Simplicity*) emphasized karma (in the sense of ethical behaviour) and preventive medicine; for example, not eating to capacity led to rewards, while unethical behaviour and over-indulgence led to retribution.

The *Tao Te Ching* talks about the five colours making the eyes blind, the five notes making the ears deaf, and the five tastes injuring the mouth. Thus a meditation place should be clean, and not too bright; it should be private, tranquil and well aired. Often Taoist communities abstain from meat, alcohol and strong flavours, although certain drugs are held to purify the body, and lead to serenity as a preparation for meditation. Many communities such as the Complete Reality School advocated celibacy, although others consider that complete celibacy is undesirable as it causes anxiety, making meditation difficult. In certain types of Chinese martial arts training, including Tai Chi Nei Kung, sexual abstinence for a period of 100 days is advocated for men.

In 2000 I asked a Taoist priest on Wudang Mountain if they (his brethren) ate meat. He said, 'Some of us do, some of us don't.' I then asked if they drank alcohol. He said, 'Some of us do, some of us don't.' Finally I asked if they had sexual congress with women. You can guess the reply.

It is clear that aspects of TCC, particularly the solo practice of forms and Nei Kung, do have both Internal Alchemy and meditation elements that enhance the martial, therapeutic and spiritual development of the practitioner. In Part II through the medium of the TCC Classics we will identify and analyse these elements in detail.

5 Classics in Chinese Culture

The most famous Chinese philosophical works to use the term '*Jing/Ching*' (Classic) in the title are the *Book of Changes* (*Yi Jing/I Ching*) and *The Classic of the Way and Virtue* (*Dao De Jing/Tao Te Ching*). These books influenced the composition of the TCC Classics, so the use of this term as a collective noun for the five major TCC texts has a certain symbolic importance. Philosophical classics were not written for, nor did the authors expect them to be applied by, the man in the street: they were aimed at the ruling élite.

Classical Chinese philosophical texts are notoriously cryptic and ambiguous, so later thinkers wrote commentaries to try to explain them. Many commentaries contain political bias, interpreting the text to give ancient authority to the political ideas supported by the author of the commentary. There are also different versions of many classical Chinese texts because, over the years, not only have scholars made mistakes in their transcription, but also deliberate interpolations and extrapolations. This is as true of ancient texts as it is of the TCC Classics.

The *Tao Te Ching* (*Canon of the Way and of Virtue*) was traditionally said to have been written by one Li Er, nicknamed 'Lao Tzu' (the Old Boy/Man), in the fifth century BC. Most experts reject this tradition and believe it to have been written sometime in the fourth century BC, and not necessarily by someone with the nickname 'Old Boy'. Different versions of the *Tao Te Ching* existed as early as 168BC, as evidenced by the finds at Han Tomb No.3 in the village of Ma Wang Düi in Hunan Province, where two versions were discovered in 1973 (one of the charts found in the tomb illustrates the *Dao Yin* exercises mentioned earlier). Not only were these some of the earliest known versions of the *Tao Te Ching*, differing in a number of respects from later versions, but also one of the two versions had the *Tao* and the *Te* sections in reverse order.

Internal Alchemy Classics

The sinologist Arthur Waley identified the first use of the term *Nei Dan* (Internal Cinnabar/Alchemy) in reference to hygienic exercise designed to promote health and tranquillity, as occurring in a Chan Buddhist text of AD565. Chinese Internal Alchemy practice has a documented history of well over 2,000 years. Though developed for health and longevity, it sometimes involved sexual practices aimed at producing an inner elixir.

In his ground-breaking work *Science and Civilisation in China* Volume V, No. 5 Joseph Needham publishes a list of dozens of Chinese treatises on Internal Alchemy, dating from the Han dynasty (205BC–AD220) onwards. One of the best known of these is the *Muscle Change Classic* (*Yi Jin Jing/I Chin Ching*). This illustrated work depicts simple hygienic exercises, said to be based on those shown by Bodhidharma in the sixth century AD to

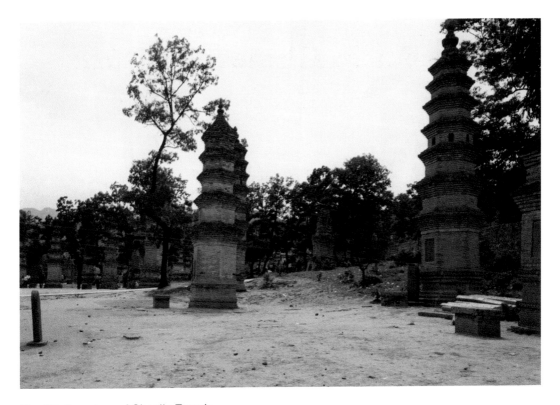

Fig. 20 Cemetery of Shaolin Temple.

monks in the Shaolin Temple to strengthen the body and as an aid to meditation. The Chan School was much influenced by (and in turn influenced) Taoism, especially the Complete Reality School.

Taoist mystical and meditation texts, such as *Nei Ye* (*Inner Training*) (c. 350BC) and the thirteenth-century Complete Reality/Truth school text, *Zhong He Ji* (*Book of Balance and Harmony*), also had a strong influence on the development of Internal Alchemy and meditation training. The exercises shown in these manuals had a major influence on the health aspects of TCC, and the terminology used in the TCC Classics shows that Tai Chi masters incorporated many ideas from Internal Alchemy into the theory of TCC.

Martial Arts Classics

Chuan Ching/Quan Jing means *Classic of Boxing*, and is the name of the best known text on Chinese martial arts. Though there may have been more than one *Classic of Boxing*, by far the most famous is attributed to Ming dynasty General Qi Ji-guang (1528– 87). There are thirty-two named martial postures, each with one illustration of a bare-chested boxer in Ming garb, and with four lines of poetic instruction on how to do the technique in a fighting situation. The thirty-two postures are eclectic, and presumably drawn from the nineteen different boxing methods that Qi mentions in the preface.

The names of nearly all the techniques of the *Classic of Boxing* exist in Chen-style TCC.

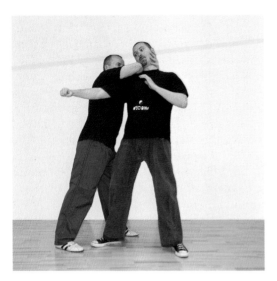

Fig. 21 Tiger Embraces Head.

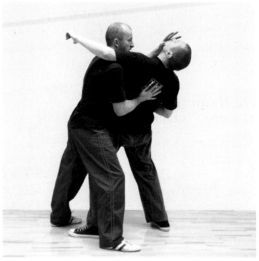

Fig. 23 Pat the Horse High.

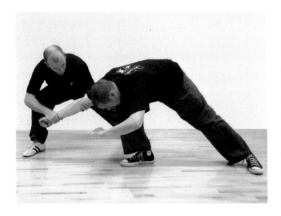

Fig. 22 Low Style.

Fewer named techniques are found in Yang lineage systems, but the poems mention other techniques that can be so found, such as Tiger Embraces Head and Low Style (sometimes called Snake Creeps Down). There are other references exactly matching TCC theory, such as the ditty explaining Pat the Horse High: 'In advancing, attacking, retreating and dodging, weakness becomes strength…'

The *Classic of Boxing* illustrates and explains how to use specific martial techniques. There are no health, meditative or philosophical elements, so the approach is quite different to that of the TCC Classics. These writings are an interesting combination of subtlety and crudity. It is the sort of thing military conscripts can be trained to do in a short period of time. However, it gives a historical perspective to many elements of Chinese martial arts in general, and of TCC in particular.

Many Chinese martial arts had secret manuals, written in a recondite manner and passed down to a chosen few but, for secrecy, oral transmission was more effective. The best work I have read on Chinese martial arts manuals is Patrick McCarthy's *The Bible of Karate Bubishi*. *Bubishi* translates as 'Manual of Martial Preparation', and is a detailed anthology of the history, philosophy and applications, including detailed illustrations, of *Dim Mak*, of Fujian White Crane and Monkfist Boxing. I had the pleasure of meeting Mr McCarthy in Finland and seeing him in action, and it is evident that what makes his book so vivid is his own considerable ability in actually doing the Kung Fu, rather than merely talking about it.

Neijiaquan/Nei Chia Chuan Classics

The other major internal martial arts, *Xingyi-Quan/Hsing-I Chuan* (Form and Intent Boxing) and *Baguazhang* (Eight Trigram Palm), also have their Classics. The origins of these seem even more obscure than the TCC Classics, and they are not so widely known. *Baguazhang* Classics consist of a multitude of short mnemonic texts. Nevertheless, there is a similarity in language – duality, Internal Alchemy and Taoist philosophy – to that found in the TCC Classics. *Xing Yi* Classics even include a Seven Stars Song, Tai Chi Song and a Wu Chi Song, while *Baguazhang* Classics mention Tai Chi techniques such as Single Whip and concepts such as *Sui* (following).

Chang Nai Zou and the TCC Classics

In recent years much has been made about similar or sometimes identical phrases appearing in the TCC Classics, in particular Classics 2 and 5, and the writings of Chang Nai Zou (AD1724–1783?), a teacher of eclectic martial arts based in Henan Province between the Northern Shaolin Temple and Chenjiagou, the Chen family village. At this time, under Emperor Qianlong, martial arts practice was proscribed and books about it were burned, hence Chang's writings could only be circulated amongst disciples. They were only published after the 1911 revolution, and were then used to train local militia. There is some doubt about how much interpolation and extrapolation has been done by persons other than Chang.

In his *Scholar Boxer*, Marnix Wells identifies many similarities between Chang's art and the *Classic of Boxing*, but also TCC. Names of techniques such as Golden Cockerel on One Leg, Seven Stars, Cross Hands, Single Whip, Ride the Tiger, Draw the Bow, Tiger Embraces Head all exist in Chang's art, in the *Classic of Boxing* and in TCC, though the postures and applications differ. Some techniques of Chang's are also similar to some TCC techniques, though they have different names. I witnessed demonstrations of Chang Nai-zhou's family boxing in 2007 by Master Liu Yiming, and discussed the connections between it and TCC, both with him and with Marnix.

There are more differences than similarities, and the differences are striking. Unlike TCC, in many of Chang's illustrations and Master Liu's postures, the centre line between the crown of the head and the coccyx is broken, with the head tilted up or down and with raised shoulders. The Chang texts talk about distending the nostrils, opening the lips and on exhalation making the sound '*Ha*'. This last is an onomatopoeic name of one of two mythical marshals from the Shang dynasty, the other being '*Heng*'. There is, however, an obscure reference in the twenty-fourth of forty texts (of which more later) published by Wu Gung-zao in 1980 of using '*Ha*' in one breath.

Chang's whole approach is very unlike TCC; there are many Buddhist references in the Chang text, suggesting influences from the nearby Shaolin Temple. Though weights are used for resistance training in some TCC schools, including my own, the Chang illustrations show the boxer wearing what appear to be bangles. Heavy metal bangles are often used in external martial arts for arm conditioning.

Professor Douglas Wile in *Lost Tai-chi Classics of the Late Ch'ing Dynasty* makes much of many phrases in Chang's writings that are

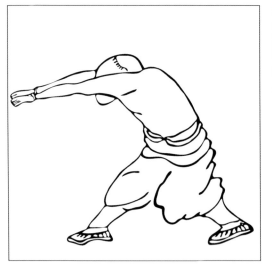 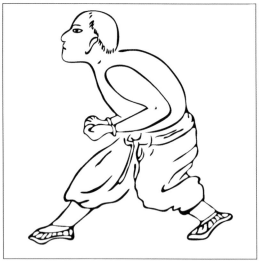

Figs 24 and 25 Illustrations of Chang Nai-zhou Boxing. Note the bangles and bent postures.

similar, or identical to material found in the TCC Classics. Chang was a teacher of eclectic boxing, so it would not be surprising if he had come across what we now call Tai Chi Chuan and borrowed ideas from it, given the time and location in which he was operating.

Even if there is a connection between Chang's art and TCC, it is strange, given that he was active in the mid-eighteenth century in the vicinity of the Chen village,

that the TCC Classics (except for Classic 5, of which the Chens have short four- and six-line versions) seem to have been unknown to the Chens; neither does Chang seem to have been much influenced by them. This suggests contact between Chang and martial artists doing something akin to TCC, who were not members of the Chen clan.

In the next section we will examine the TCC Classics in detail.

PART II
THE TAI CHI CHUAN CLASSICS

6 The Tai Chi Chuan Classics

The *Tai Chi Chuan Ching/Taijiquan Jing* (TCC Classics) consist of only five texts, which contain many, but not all, of the most important principles and concepts of the art, and are the main source of our universal truths for the modern martial artist. The theory in the Classics was developed through martial, therapeutic, alchemical and meditative practice. It is these five texts more than any others that are reproduced or quoted in books on the art, so they are the most valuable written sources of TCC theory, and deserving of the name 'Tai Chi Chuan Classics'. They are:

1. The Tai Chi Chuan Discourse – *Tai Chi Chuan Lun*
2. The Canon of Tai Chi Chuan – *Tai Chi Chuan Ching*
3. Interpretation of the Practice of the Thirteen Tactics – *Shi San Shi Xing Gong Xin Jie*
4. Song of the Thirteen Tactics – *Shi San Shi Ge*
5. The Fighter's Song (Song of Striking Hands) – *Da Shou Ge*

Some books call Classic 1 by the name of Classic 2 and vice versa, or give them in a different order, but the format given above is the way I learned them, and the content of the texts is more important than the titles.

The character for 'Classic' is romanized *Jing/Ching*. It is the general term used to refer to these five writings, as well as the term I have translated as 'Canon' in respect of the title of the second text. Other terms such as '*Jue*' (formula) are used to refer to writings added as postscripts to Texts 3, 4 and 5. I will deal with the five Classics individually after setting out the background to the texts and translations.

These texts are not a coherent or logical body of work. There are numerous phrases or concepts from one text being reproduced in another. There are differences in emphasis: the Fighter's Song is concerned solely with practical fighting concepts using ideas drawn from Sun Tzu's *Art of War*, while the other texts all contain ideas about movement and health as well as fighting concepts. Some ideas from Neo-Confucian and Taoist philosophy also occur in the texts, as well as references to Internal Alchemy, Chinese philosophy, religion and divination.

All this suggests that the Classics were written by more than one person, and possibly at different periods in the evolution of TCC. Be aware, the Classics are not the sum repository of human wisdom on the subject of TCC, nor, as you will perceive from the commentaries, do I agree with every word written by the author/s.

Discovery and Authorship of the TCC Classics

A century after Chang Naizhou's heyday, 1852 was a significant year. It was the year Yang Lu-chan left Yongnian and his students, the three Wu brothers, to go to teach in Beijing. Just after this, and also in 1852, Wu Yu-xiang goes to find Yang's master, Chen Chang-xing (one year before Chen's death), but ends up at the nearby Zhao Bao village where he trains under Chen Qing-ping for a month, 'learning all his secrets'.

Many books relate how, in 1852, the five major TCC Classics turn up in a salt store in Wu Yang County, Henan, where Yang's student, Wu Cheng-qing, happens to be the local magistrate. Research by Barbara Davis, in her 2004 book *The Taijiquan Classics*, now casts doubt on this tale because of problems with the dates. At that time and well into

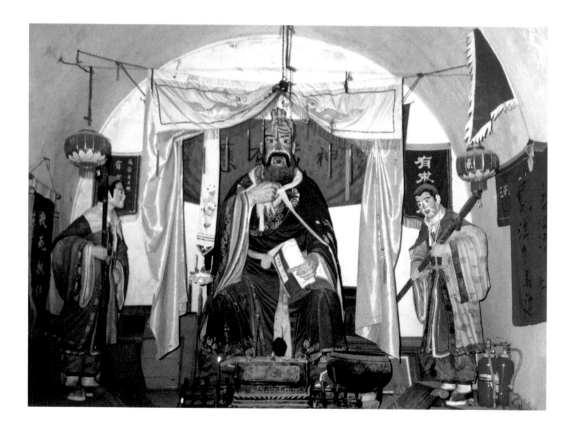

Fig. 26 Statue of Chang San-feng, Golden Pavilion Temple, Baoji.

the twentieth century, the Chinese used the reign name and year of the emperor and the lunar calendar to give the date. The Western calendar was then introduced, and increased the confusion. Mistakes were often made both with emperor names and years by many people, not least historians.

Li Yi-yu, nephew of the Wu brothers, purportedly wrote a preface to a version of most of the five Classics material with other texts in the 1880s, in which he refers to Yang Lu-chan as a 'certain Yang'. There is some doubt about the provenance of the writings: often the authorship of classical Chinese writings would be ascribed to some eminent individual to give them authority.

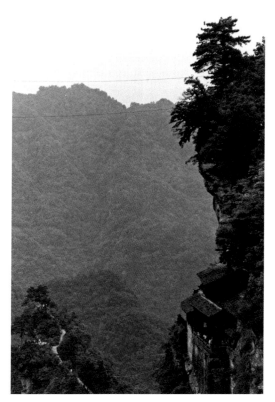

Fig. 27 Wudang Mountain, temples on the Southern Cliff.

Classic 1 (TCC Discourse) is often attributed to Chang San-feng, the Taoist hermit, who lived sometime around the fourteenth century AD and who is recognized by many Yang lineage schools as the founder of TCC. Given the definite influences in the names of certain Tai Chi Nei Kung postures, in terminology and in meditative practice from the Complete Reality School (of which Chang was a member) on TCC, it is a possibility.

Classic 2 (Canon of TCC) is most often attributed to Wang Zong-yue, who was active as a teacher and scholar around Kaifeng in 1791 and Luoyang in 1795. These localities are both in Henan Province and relatively near to the Chen village, so it is possible (as the Yang lineages mostly claim) that Wang taught TCC to Jiang Fa, who passed it on to Chen Chang-xing, teacher of Yang Lu-chan.

Sometimes Classics 3, 4 and 5 (Interpretation of the Practice of The Thirteen Tactics; Song of the Thirteen Tactics; and the Fighter's Song) are also attributed to Wang or sometimes to Yang Lu-chan's student, Wu Yu-xiang, or someone else entirely, such as Yang Lu-chan himself; no proof exists one way or the other. This would also explain why the Chens and the Yangs do not claim to have written any of the TCC Classics. Some authors attribute at least Classics 2 to 5, and possibly all five, to Wang. Concepts are repeated in different Classics and there are differences in style and content, all of which suggests that the five major TCC Classics are the work of more than one author. In the versions of the Classics in this book, both 3 and 5 end with interpolations that are most likely the work of later masters, as they are not to be found in every version of the said Classics.

There are numerous works dating from the Qing dynasty attributed to Chang San-feng, but which were actually produced by spirit writing (*Fu Qi*), a process similar to using the ouija board. The spirit world is contacted and the spirit responds through the medium, writing characters on sand contained in a planchette. The resulting writings are then interpreted by the medium and attributed to the spirit in question.

In Chapter 2 of Chao Pi-chen's (born AD1860) *Secrets of Cultivation of Essential Nature and Eternal Life*, Chao quotes Chang San-feng as encouraging old people indulging in sexual Internal Alchemy practice to masturbate to arouse the genital organ. By the time the book was published Chang had become known as the founder of TCC, and was also a cult figure amongst Taoists. Chao's quote is dubious, though Chang did have a reputation as an alchemist. Other works were also attributed to Chang San-feng through the medium of spirit writing, so why not the Classics? Alternatively a later master may simply have attributed the Classics to Chang San-feng and Wang Zong-yue to give them greater authority.

Transmission of the TCC Classics

After receiving TCC instruction from his uncle, Cheng Wing-kwong, in Hong Kong during World War II, my teacher, Cheng Tin-hung, became a disciple of Qi Min-xuan, from Hebei Dao in Henan Province. After Cheng went through '*Bai Shi*' (the ritual initiation where students 'enter the door' to become disciples), Qi made him memorize the TCC Classics by chanting them when practising the Tai Chi Nei Kung.

This method of learning classical texts is common in Chinese culture, and it is likely that for many generations this was how the Classics were handed down until TCC went public in the early twentieth century. Oral transmission had the dual advantages of preventing 'secret knowledge' being passed on to outsiders, while also being an ideal method for adepts to learn the theory. With no written version of the Classics to fall back on, a practitioner had to rely on the oral version, so it is easy to add or leave out characters or to confuse similar-sounding characters or intonation from different dialects. On the written side it is also easy to insert a similar-looking or sounding character, or for a printer to 'correct' or misread a handwritten text. Some terms in the TCC Classics such as '*Peng*' and '*Lu*' cannot be found in dictionaries and were either wrongly transcribed, or were specially invented technical terms.

Oral transmission is still used to teach important aspects of the art, other than the TCC Classics. My teacher taught me many things on a one-to-one basis, such as Six Secret Words, invaluable in self-defence. Another example is a mantra for composing the mind before some serious undertaking. Neither is to be found in any text on TCC. Nowadays many TCC students follow and attempt to copy the teacher's movements, and there is usually little explanation. Such students can get something out of a study of the Classics, but the more limited their exposure to the varied elements in TCC, the more limited will be their ability to comprehend the Classics and to understand what they are doing.

Interpretation of the TCC Classics

The technical nature of much of the content of the TCC Classics has led to two major developments. Firstly, the Classics are often translated to fit the knowledge of the translator, who often ignores or fails to explain concepts (if he has no fighting experience he is unlikely to make sense of the Fighter's Song), and over-emphasizes other concepts with which he is familiar. Secondly, people changed their TCC to fit their (often perverse) interpretations of concepts in the Classics, so that their art became quite different from that of their masters. We can compare the postures of well known masters such as Wu Gong-yi and his father, Wu Jian-quan, or those of Cheng Man-ching with his main teacher, Yang Cheng-fu. They are not the same, and yet teachers in these lineages would claim that they are practising traditional TCC and use the TCC Classics for support. So we have a paradox, where the Classics as they are understood by an individual affect that individual's TCC, and that individual's knowledge of TCC limits his ability to understand the Classics.

Some translations are less than honest and are flowery and vague, using the same general term such as 'energy' to explain different concepts such as '*Qi*' and '*Jin*'. The jargon used in the original Chinese texts and in many translations makes the Classics an impenetrable jungle for the average martial artist. In the translations therefore, I have used the romanized version of key Chinese technical terms that constantly recur, and have explained the meaning of these terms in the commentaries. I have included an introduction and commentary to each Classic, and have explained the key concepts with pictures and diagrams. Because I've made my translation as close to the original Chinese as possible, sometimes the English version may not seem felicitously worded. However, the Classics are decoded by the commentaries and illustrations, and understood through practice.

The TCC Classics are aimed at those who are at a level beyond that of the beginner or dilettante. The vast majority of practitioners don't have the knowledge to interpret and follow the fascinating and insightful material in the TCC Classics, which can, like philosophical classics, be of use to anyone who has the resolve to apply them. Incorrect understanding leads to incorrect practice.

This explanation of the TCC Classics aims to improve the practice and understanding of even novice martial artists. Understanding

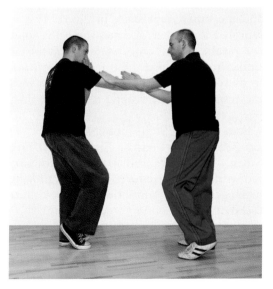 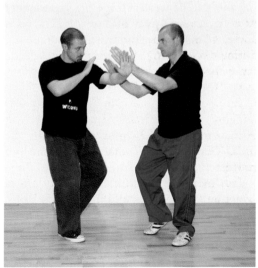

Figs 28 and 29 Seven Star Step.

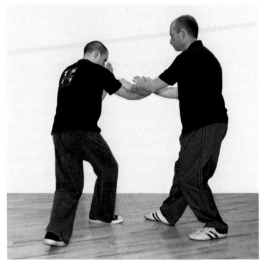
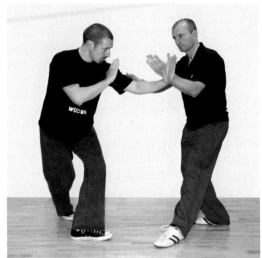

Figs 30 and 31 Nine Palace Step.

the theory goes hand in hand with improvements in practice, but only insofar as theory and practice are related. If there is no partner work then martial understanding will be limited; if there is no practice of Internal Alchemy beyond the form, this understanding will also be weak. I hope my experiences as a fighter and as a teacher of TCC as a complete martial, meditative and therapeutic exercise system make this a practical guide for every martial artist.

TCC Footwork

A recurring theme helpful in analyzing the TCC Classics is footwork. Apart from foot movements in the forms, there are three major methods of TCC footwork, all of which are also major Pushing hands drills. They include Seven Star Step, Nine Palace Step and Four Corner Step, which is colloquially known as Great Diversion (*Da Lu*).

Seven Star Step is a zig-zag stepping pattern where one partner steps forwards with a push, and the other steps back to divert. This is repeated a number of times, then the roles are reversed. Seven Star Step is also found in other internal martial arts.

Nine Palace Step is a stepping pattern where one partner steps across with a push, and the other steps back to divert. This is repeated a number of times, then the roles are reversed. The cross step or traverse is similar to *Baguazhang* and fencing footwork to move around a technique or to spin with the response when dealing with more than one opponent.

Four Corner Step – best known as *Da Lu* (Great Diversion) or Eight Gates, Five Steps – is an advanced method of training footwork with a partner while employing locking, butting, uprooting and spiralling techniques.

In most applications we will use footwork so the angle of techniques will often be different from that found in the form. Failure to use footwork will often lead to brute force being used against brute force.

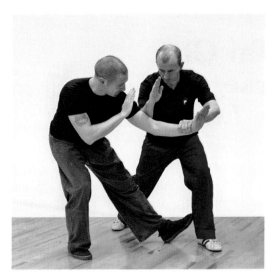

Versions of the Tai Chi Chuan Classics

The versions of the Classics on which my translation is based are from *Statement of Requirements of Tai Chi Chuan (Tai Chi Chuan Shu Yao)* by Cheng Tin-hung, and are the fullest versions I could find. Other versions tend to be shorter, probably because people left out what they did not understand or could not remember from the oral tradition.

Fig. 32 Four Corner Step, also known as *Da Lu* or 8 Gates, 5 Steps.

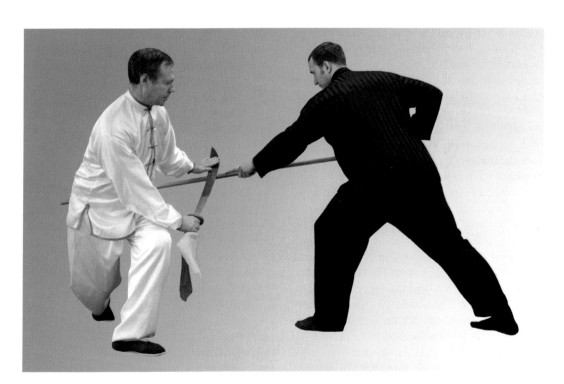

Author demonstrates Lying Fish, using Nine Palace Step.

7 Classic 1: The Tai Chi Chuan Discourse (*Tai Chi Chuan Lun*)

There is some disagreement about the titles of Classics 1 and 2: some authorities have *Tai Chi Chuan Ching* (The Canon of Tai Chi Chuan) as the title for Classic 1, and *Tai Chi Chuan Lun* for Classic 2. I have given the titles as I was taught them; the content is more important than the title.

The term *Lun* is found in *Lun Yu*, the Analects of Confucius, which are discourses of the master on how to conduct oneself within a moral and social context. The *Tai Chi Chuan Lun* likewise instructs us how to conduct ourselves within a physical and, more particularly, a martial context. Lao Tzu said:

> …some things lead, some follow;
> Some are strong, some weak;
> Some destroy, some are destroyed,
> Hence the sage avoids excess…
> (*Tao Te Ching* Ch. 29)

This Classic is often attributed to the Taoist hermit, Chang San-feng (c. fourteenth century), but there is no proof for this, one way or the other. It contains many references to duality: up and down, left and right, forwards and back, bumps and hollows, extended and cut off, full and empty. Duality and change are important from a martial viewpoint, but they are also essential influences on both circulation and respiration. More succinctly, TCC practice is the complementary interaction of Yin and Yang in myriad ways.

Chuang Tzu talked of separation leading to completion, from which came dissolution – but all things, regardless of this completion and dissolution, may still be understood in their unity; not everyone appreciates this.

TCC Classic 1

*Once you move, the whole body
must be light and agile,
In particular, it must be linked together.
The Qi (vital energy) should
be excited to activity,
While the Shen (spirit) must
be internally hoarded.
No place should be deficient or defective,
No place should have hollows or bumps.
No place should be cut off or overextended.
The root is in the feet;
Discharging is done by the legs,
The controlling power is in the waist,
And the appearance is in the hand and fingers.
From the feet to the legs to the waist,
All must be completely uniform and done
in one breath (literally, 'one Qi'),
Whether stepping forward or moving back.
This will result in good timing
and correct movements.
If in certain places good timing and
correct movement are not achieved,
Body movements become
arbitrary and disordered.
This sickness must be sought
in the waist and leg.*

Above and below, forward and back,
left and right are all like this.
In general this is controlled by the
Yi (intent) and not externally.
If there is up, immediately there is down;
If there is forward, immediately there is back;
If there is left, immediately there is right.
If the Yi is to go up,
The Yi to go down is there immediately.
Or, if you raise something up,
Then there is the Yi to smash it
down with increased force.
In this way its roots will be severed
And destruction will be swift and beyond doubt.
Void and substantial must be clearly distinguished.
Each place of course has its individual
balance of void and substantial,
Every place consists of this, one
void and substantial.
Every part of the body in turn is strung together,
Without causing the least break.
This Chang Chuan (Long Boxing),
It's like the great river, the Chang Jiang,
Surging and flowing, without interruption.
Of the Thirteen Tactics,
Peng, Lu, Ji, An, Cai, Lie, Zhou and Kao;
They are the Eight Trigrams.
Step Forwards, Move Back, Face Left,
Look Right and Centrally Stable;
These are the Five Elements.
Peng, Lu, Ji and An,
Are the trigrams Chien, Kun, Kan,
Li, the four cardinal points.
Cai, Lie, Zhou and Kao
Are the trigrams Sun, Chen,
Tui, Ken, the four corners.
Step Forwards, Move Back, Face Left,
Look Right and Centrally Stable;
Are Metal, Wood, Water, Fire and Earth.

Commentary

Once you move, the whole body
must be light and agile,
In particular, it must be linked together.

If we are tense or move in an unco-ordinated manner, the balance, speed and smoothness of our technique will be adversely affected. This applies to self-defence and to forms equally. If we are light and agile we can change direction more quickly. At the same time there is a paradoxical requirement that in any stance at least one foot, and sometimes both feet are rooted to the ground. In being rooted the body and limbs are like a bamboo plant, able to sway easily in harmony with the elements. The constant shifting of weight, combined with centre line flexion and rotation as we move in any direction, creates agility.

TCC hand forms are normally practised slowly and softly to develop relaxation; this also lets us feel the technique. Pushing hands drills such as Nine Palace Step and Seven Star Step train footwork, timing and distance, which enables the body to be 'light and agile'. The linking together, or co-ordination, is trained in the moving Tai Chi Nei Kung exercises and in pushing hands drills such as Single Hand and Four Directions.

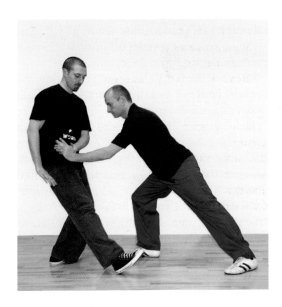

Fig. 33 Single Hand Pushing hands.

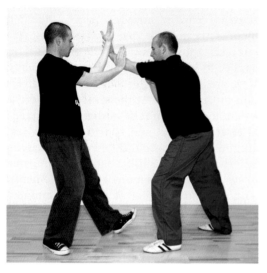 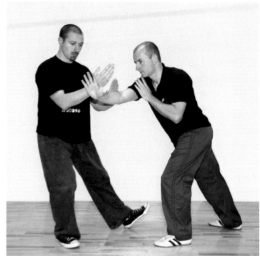

Figs 34 and 35 Four Directions pushing hands.

The Qi (vital energy) should
be excited to activity,
While the Shen (spirit) must
be internally hoarded.

Qi and *Shen* together with *Jing* are the three interactive treasures of the Taoist alchemists, and are key concepts in traditional Chinese medicine and *Qi Gong*.

I have rendered *Qi* as 'vital energy' in the present context, but this is not an adequate explanation of the concept. The character represents rice being cooked in a pot and giving off vapour, so there is the idea of the alchemical change beloved by Taoists. *Qi* is many different things: there is *Qi* all around us; the air is *Qi*. The oxygen that we extract from the air is *Qi*. The oxygen, transported by haemoglobin, which is delivered from the lungs to the tissues of the body, is *Qi*. The carbon dioxide and methane gas discharged from various orifices are also examples of *Qi*. 'Vital energy' seems the best choice of translation, despite its limitations.

The character *Shen* represents, on the left, the sky and the heavenly bodies, and on the right, two hands extending a rope, giving the idea of expansion. The combination has man reaching for the stars to receive the will of Heaven, so perhaps 'spirit' is the best translation in the present context.

The third treasure, *Jing*, means 'vital essence', such as seminal fluid and vaginal secretions. The left of the character depicts

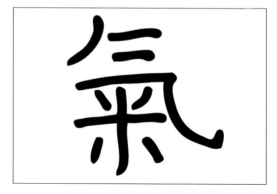

Fig. 36 Character for *Qi*.

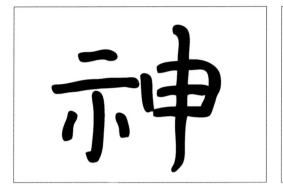

Fig. 37 Character for *Shen*.

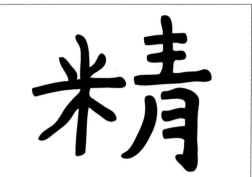

Fig. 38 Character for *Jing*.

the rice plant, while on the right the upper part means 'to give birth', and the lower represents the colour of plants. Without a good supply of *Qi* the essence would be lacking and the *Shen* would not be at ease. If the *Shen* were not tranquil, the breathing would be adversely affected, and the ability to produce or retain *Jing* would be adversely affected.

Lao Tzu talks about how 'Within it (the way) there is an essence (*Jing*). This essence is quite genuine, and within it is something that can be tested' (*Tao Te Ching* Ch. 21).

Taoists believe sickness arises when there is a lack, an excess, or a blockage of *Qi* or *Jing*. Many people, particularly those with sedentary life styles and the elderly, suffer from poor respiration and circulation, but it is possible to increase the respiration and stimulate the circulation by exercise. This requires full movements involving sinking and raising, contracting and expanding; thus *Qi* can be said to be 'excited to activity'. The character '*Gu*', which I have rendered as 'excited', has the main meaning of 'drum' and by extension 'swelling' or 'rousing'. Here it emphasizes the effect caused by the *Qi* in the abdominal area, particularly around the *Dan Tian*. '*Dang*', which I have rendered as 'activity', can also mean 'a bathtub', so the

essence is of water moving about as it does when one is bathing. This is an exaggerated way of saying that the *Qi* should be active rather than stagnant, and this activity is generated by the liveliness of the movements. However, Lao Tzu also said, 'For the mind to send the *Qi* is called violence' (*Tao Te Ching* Ch. 55). So *Qi* and *Jing* should develop naturally and not be forced.

Smooth and co-ordinated movement ensures that the *Shen* is calm and therefore the concentration is good, whether in soft practice or in fighting. This also means that TCC practitioners rarely use the grimaces and facial contortions to be seen in Kung Fu movies. However, it does not mean that we are devoid of emotion or intent when fighting.

No place should be deficient or defective,
No place should have hollows or bumps.
No place should be cut off or overextended.

Deficient or defective moves occur where, for example, we raise the hand to defend but fail to make a complementary body movement, or where we strike an opponent, but fail to use body force. In defence we try to add to the opponent's force, rather than opposing it.

49

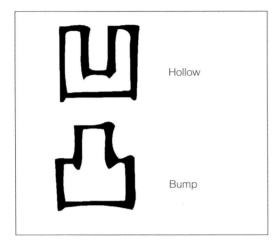

Fig. 39 Chinese characters meaning 'hollow' and 'bump'.

The Chinese characters for hollows and bumps are pictographs. If we don't extend the arms sufficiently in, say, Single Whip, a hollow is created at the elbow joint; if the backside is sticking out, a bump is created.

Techniques such as this should be extended so that the elbow joint is just short of being locked; there is Yin within Yang and Yang within Yin in all techniques. This is a physical way of expressing the dot of Yang in Yin and the dot of Yin in Yang in the Tai Chi symbol. Bumps indicate localized tension, as where the shoulders or back are hunched when we perform an arm movement.

Many practitioners run techniques together by 'cutting off' – that is, failing to finish one movement before starting the next, or they overextend their techniques. In a front stance, we go sufficiently far forwards that the front knee extends over, but not beyond, the toes of the front foot. The weight is therefore mainly on this foot; only when we get this far forwards do we start to move back, turn or step forwards. Going further forwards will cause us to 'uproot' ourselves and can cause knee damage, especially amongst older practitioners. The key lies in correct weight transference. Many novices overextend by either locking the elbow joint or throwing forwards

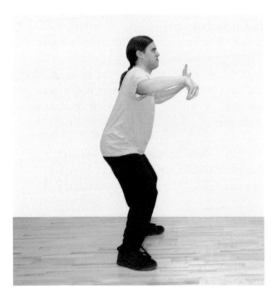
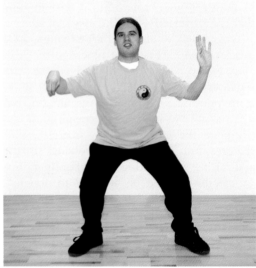

Figs 40 and 41 Single Whip bad posture.

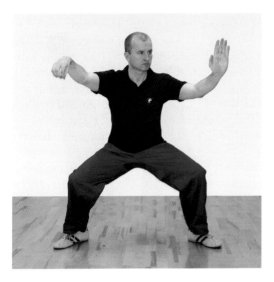

Fig. 42 Single Whip correct posture.

the shoulder of the arm when delivering a forward strike or thrust. If we do this and miss the target, we are very vulnerable; even if we hit, it is difficult to recover. The object in self-defence is not to hit the opponent as hard as we can, but to hit in a safe and secure way, so that we are able to follow up or change direction as circumstances dictate.

This concept was familiar to Medieval and Renaissance martial artists and is known as the principle of recovery. In both Chinese and European sword traditions there are specific techniques employed to make a recovery after failing with a first move.

Chuang Tzu has a story about a wheelwright who explains that in making a wheel, if he proceeds gently, the workmanship is not strong; but if he proceeds violently, it is wearisome and the joinings don't fit. If the movement of his hands is neither gentle nor violent, his idea is realized. It is the same when practising martial arts.

The root is in the feet;
Discharging is done by the legs.
The controlling power is in the waist,
And the appearance is in the hand
and fingers.

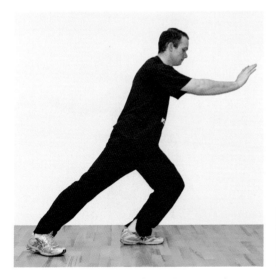

Fig. 43 As if Shutting a Door. Incorrect knee position, leading to overextending the upper body.

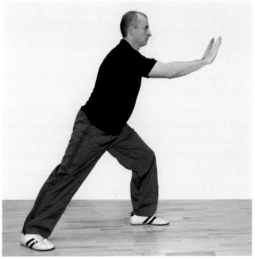

Fig. 44 As if Shutting a Door. Correct posture.

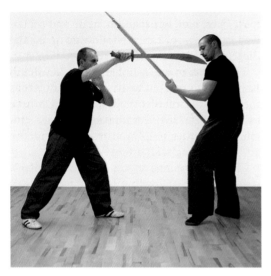

Fig. 45 Sabre technique, Climb Mountain to look into Distance, is deflected by spearman.

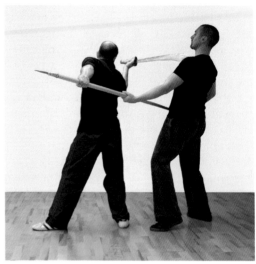

Fig. 46 Sabre man recovers with spin into sabre technique, *Peng* spreads Wings.

Lao Tzu tells us 'What is firmly rooted cannot be pulled out, what is tightly embraced will not slip loose.' (*Tao Te Ching*, Ch. 54).

When we need to root the feet we do so by sinking, thereby lowering the centre of gravity; thus the feet root us to the ground like a plant, while the body moves freely – like the said plant being blown by the wind. Beginners usually concentrate on what the teacher is doing with his hands, and fail to see that the discharging power or momentum is coming from the feet through the legs to the waist, and finally to the hands and arms. Discharge (*Fa*) is also a reference to *Fa Jin*, which is to emit force.

When pushing off the rear foot, the rear leg straightens, pushing the weight forwards on to the front leg; at the same time the waist (centre line) turns as in 'Step Up, Deflect, Parry and Punch', when we start to deliver the punch. Beginners tend to concentrate on the punch, and fail to notice the other parts of the process; as a result they often transfer their weight forwards before the technique has been delivered, rather than with the technique. The same concept applies when using a downward pull to uproot the opponent, in that the legs bend at the knee to effect a sudden drop in our centre of gravity; the whole bodyweight is involved in the technique.

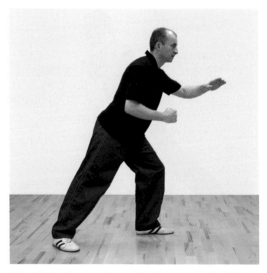

Fig. 47 Bad technique. The legs have finished, but the arms are still travelling.

This problem can be remedied by pushing hands and Tai Chi Nei Kung training, where we repeat the same movements many times, while discharging with the legs and turning the centre line and hence the waist, hips, shoulders and legs. Some practitioners try to distinguish between hips and waist; others try to insist that as only the waist is mentioned, only the waist should turn. This is mere sophism: everything turns when there is a rotation of the central line – the spinal column.

From the feet to the legs to the waist,
All must be completely uniform and done
in one breath (literally, 'one Qi'),
Whether stepping forwards or moving back.
This will result in good timing
and correct movements.
If in certain places good timing and
correct movement are not achieved,
Body movements become arbitrary and disordered.
This sickness must be sought
in the waist and leg.
Above and below, forward and back,
left and right are all like this.
In general this is controlled by the
Yi (intent) and not externally.

TCC requires total body movement rather than localized or unco-ordinated movement. All parts of the body should therefore start and finish a technique together. This skill can be trained in pushing hands and application drills using complementary body movement: if your partner goes forwards, you go back, and vice versa; this going forwards or back can involve weight transference alone, or stepping and weight transference together. The forms train all this only to a limited degree; for the elements of timing, distance and angle to be correct, there is no substitute for partner work.

I showed this excerpt from the Classics to an experienced German TCC exponent who expressed amazement that physicality was emphasized, rather than focusing on the *Dan Tian* (Cinnabar Field). This confusion is common, as the Classics go back and forth between Internal Alchemy and martial arts.

I have translated '*Yi Qi*' as 'done in one breath', meaning simultaneously and not ponderously. Lao Tzu remarked that in action it is timeliness that matters. Most people end up getting hurt in a fight because either they freeze and fail to react, or they react too late: hence the importance of drills to train reflex action.

The last two lines emphasize the use of the intent or focused thought to control the movements, no matter in what direction, so that we overcome an opponent with technique and don't merely react to his attacks.

If there is up, immediately there is down;
If there is forwards, immediately there is back;
If there is left, immediately there is right.
If the Yi is to go up,
The Yi to go down immediately is there.
Or, if you raise something up,

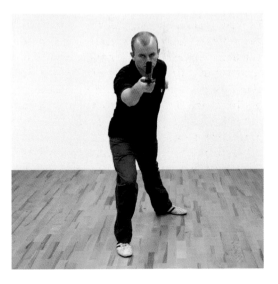

Fig. 48 Pierce the Heart.

Then there is the Yi to smash it
down with increased force.
In this way its roots will be severed
And destruction will be swift and beyond doubt.

The *Yi* (intent) controls above and below, forwards and back, left and right, and *Yi* occurs when mind and technique combine to focus. With the sword in 'Pierce the Heart', the sword tip, our nose, front knee and centre line (spinal column) are all going in the same direction. The eyes, which show the intent, should also be looking in that direction, as that is where the force is going. This is what makes a technique decisive and penetrating.

We can look at the dualities about left and right, forwards and back, up and down, from a health and from a martial standpoint. From a health point of view, TCC forms involve constantly contrasting movements, first in one direction, then in another. This method is excellent for improving balance and co-ordination. The circulation and joint movement are also improved. By raising the hands above the head, the heart has to work harder to pump the blood through the arteries against gravity, but the blood drains easily through the veins back down to the heart. Lowering the hands has the reverse effect, making it easy for the blood to flow from the heart down through the arteries towards the hands and fingers, but making it more difficult for the blood to flow up through the veins to the heart.

A good example of raising up to smash down is using 'Raise Hands, Step Up' to duck a head punch, using the opponent's forward momentum assisted by a groin strike to raise him up over the shoulder and smash him down behind us.

The principle of total body movement applies no matter what direction we are moving in: this is the practical application of Yin Yang theory as directed by the intent. If we try to lift an opponent and he resists, then we change the force to downward directed force; if we pull him forwards and he resists, we throw him back as in 'Snake Creeps Down/Low Style'. If we divert his attack with the left hand, then it is natural to

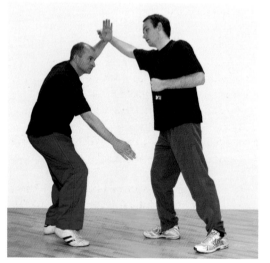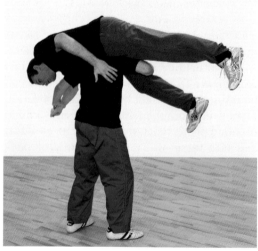

Figs 49 and 50 Raise Hands, Step Up.

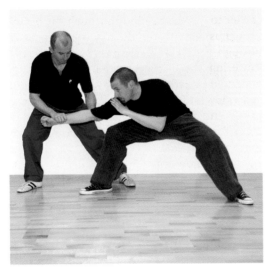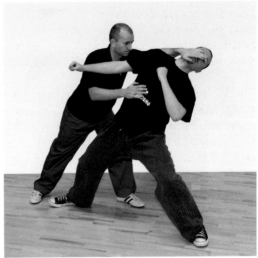

Figs 51 and 52 Snake Creeps Down.

hit him immediately with the right, as with 'Stroke the Lute'.

This is applied psychology. The opponent attacks us and wants to hurt us, therefore whatever we do, he will oppose it; thus if we exert force in one direction, he is likely to resist us. When we detect his resistance, we can use maximum force in the opposite reaction, as with 'Step Back Repulse Monkey'. This indirect method of detecting resistance and exploiting it is much more devastating, as we are exploiting the opponent's anger and adding our force to his. This skill is referred to as '*Ting Jin*': listening for force, not just with the ears, but with the whole body. '*Ting*' (listen) is referred to in Classic 4, but we are not told what to listen for. The concept of listening for force is not mentioned in any of the TCC Classics, though many principles connected with it are. I will deal with it when discussing Classic 2.

Listening ability and the ability to uproot or unbalance an opponent is trained by repetitive pushing hands drills, free pushing (whether fixed or moving step) and TCC grappling, until it becomes a natural reaction

in self-defence. The Confucian text, *The Great Learning* (*Da Xue*, written c. 200BC), states that if the root is in chaos one cannot be in order, and that knowing the root is the highest knowledge. Therefore one of the objects of severing an opponent's root is to make him vulnerable to a follow-up technique, because all he can think of at that moment is trying to keep his balance.

Void and substantial must be
clearly distinguished.
Each place of course has its individual
balance of void and substantial,
Every place consists of this, one
void and substantial.
Every part of the body in turn is strung together,
Without causing the least break.

Void means empty and can be seen as Yang. Substantial means full and can be seen as Yin. In a front stance the front foot is substantial/ full/Yin, and we normally can't step with it unless and until we shift the weight on to the other foot (or use the 'drop step'). Effectively the foot is dead – this is what makes it Yin.

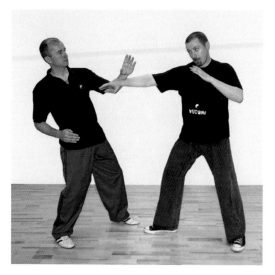

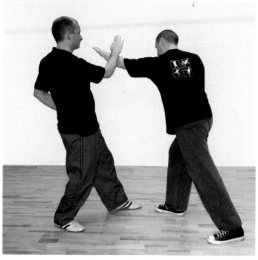

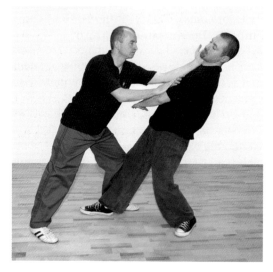

CLOCKWISE FROM TOP LEFT: Figs 53–55 Stroke the Lute.

Similarly, when in a front stance, the rear foot is void/empty/Yang, and can step easily in any direction. This potential for movement is what makes it Yang. This can be seen in the Four Directions pushing hands drill in Figs 34 and 35 (*see* page 48).

In a back stance or cat stance the rear leg is full and Yin, while the front leg is empty

and Yang for exactly the same reasons. When in a horse-riding stance the void and substantiality exists insofar as the lower body is full or Yin, while the upper body is Yang as it has the potential for movement by inclining and turning to shift the weight in another direction and into a front, back or other type of stance.

This division also applies to the hands. Normally, if one hand is striking, the other hand is ready to strike and the force is concentrated on the striking hand at the moment of impact. However, we don't just strike with the hands, but with the whole body force. In pushing hands and fighting, our choices of full and empty correspond to what the opponent does, and are guided by our intent and trained response.

Some teachers use these metaphors connecting Yin and Yang with void and substantial differently from me. Don't be too concerned with this: the main thing is to understand the difference between void and substantial. Mentally, too, there is a division of void and substantial; intending to defend automatically implies intending to counter, and vice versa. Counters can be changed if they are unsuccessful, or if the opponent resists.

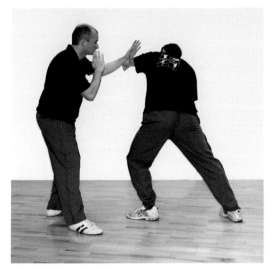

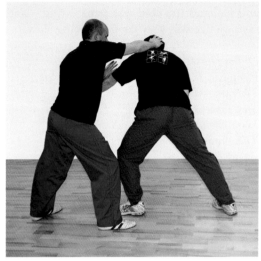

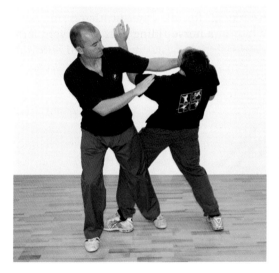

CLOCKWISE FROM TOP LEFT: Figs 56–58 Step Back Repulse Monkey.

This Chang Chuan (Long Boxing),
It's like the great river, the Chang Jiang,
Surging and flowing without interruption.

Chang Chuan is one of nineteen schools of boxing on which the *Classic of Boxing* (*Chuanching/Quanjing*) is supposedly based. The preface refers to 'The 32 techniques/ styles of *Chang Chuan* (Long Boxing) from Emperor Tai Zu (AD960–976) of the Song dynasty'. I have a book on a *Chang Chuan* form, which, though external in nature, contains techniques such as Single Whip, Heel Kick, Two Raises of the Leg and White Crane Flaps Wings: all these names are found in TCC Long Form. Here, *Chang Chuan* is used as another name for TCC. The name was derived from China's famous river, the Chang Jiang. This comparison implies that, like a river, our movements, whether in self-defence, forms or pushing hands, should flow and be continuous, using total body movement. Also, we need to spend time on long and regular practice to benefit from TCC. Just as a river changes in speed and in the nature of its flow according to the terrain and the amount of water available, so there is no one way in which, or one speed at which, we should do the form. Some movements are more demanding than others, some require greater or lesser emphasis.

TCC forms can be done in a slower, softer and internalized way, or in a more vigorous, martial way. Some years ago I visited Wudang Mountain in late December: there was snow

57

and ice, and the cold was penetrating – and my practice was very far from being slow.

Of the Thirteen Tactics,
Peng, Lu, Ji, An, Cai, Lie, Zhou and Kao;
They are the Eight Trigrams.
Step Forwards, Move Back, Face Left,
Look Right and Centrally Stable;
These are the Five Elements.

I have used the translation 'Thirteen Tactics' rather than the more common 'Thirteen Movements', because they are not just thirteen ways of moving, but eight ways of applying trained force combined with five ways of standing and stepping. They are not used in an arbitrary way, but are logical responses to an opponent's actions. 'Centrally Stable' is also sometimes translated as 'Central Equilibrium'.

Peng, Lu, Ji and An,
Are the trigrams Chien, Kun, Kan,
Li; the four cardinal points.
Cai, Lie, Zhou and Kao
Are the trigrams Sun, Chen,
Tui, Ken; the four corners.
Step Forwards, Move Back, Face Left,
Look Right and Centrally Stable;
Are Metal, Wood, Water, Fire and Earth.

There are two main arrangements of the Eight Trigrams. The Prior to Heaven arrangement was attributed to legendary emperor Fu Xi, who was also credited with inventing methods of writing, fishing and trapping. He is supposed to have lived around 2400BC, predating the writing of the original *Book of Changes* (fifteenth to eleventh century BC). This is the arrangement of the Eight Trigrams almost invariably associated with the

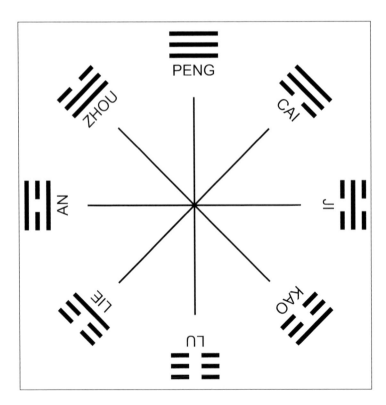

Fig. 59 Relationship of the Prior to Heaven arrangement of the Eight Trigrams and the Eight Forces.

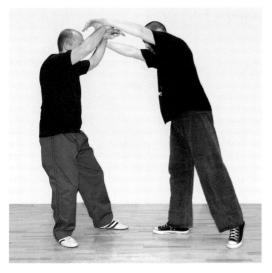
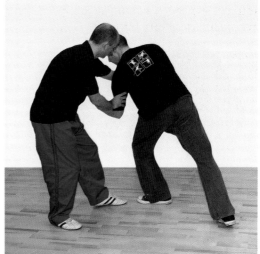
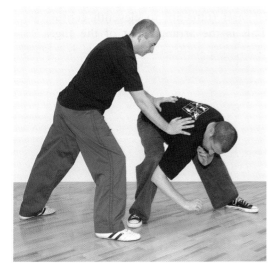
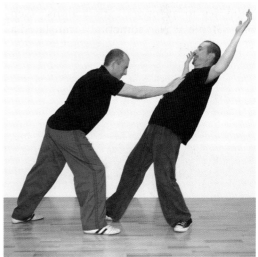

CLOCKWISE FROM TOP LEFT: Fig. 60 *Peng.* Fig. 61 *Lu.* Fig. 62 *Ji.* Fig. 63 *An.*

Eight Forces. The other major arrangement is the Post Heaven version of King Wen (Cultural/Civil), the father of King Wu (Martial) who is said to have been the founder of the Zhou dynasty (c. 1100BC).

The first essay in a series of forty writings published by the Yang and Wu families – and therefore presumably having their endorsement – gives a different relationship between the Eight Trigrams and the Eight Forces to that given in the Classics. This is, I fear, another of their many never-to-be-explained mistakes.

The main reason for identifying a particular trigram with a particular way of using force is that each force is usually directed to a specific trigram. For example, in using *Peng* our hand/s diverts the opponent's arm/s up from

59

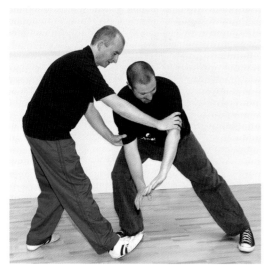
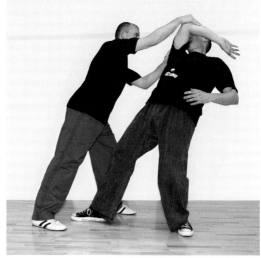
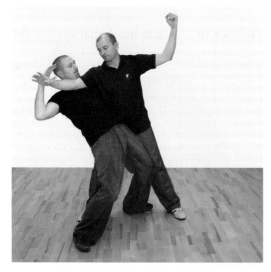
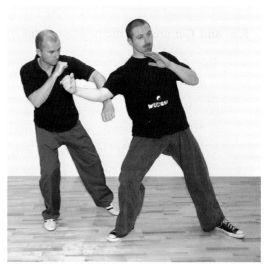

CLOCKWISE FROM TOP LEFT: Fig. 64 *Cai*. Fig. 65 *Lie*. Fig. 66 *Zhou*. Fig. 67 *Kao*.

underneath – that is, towards the trigram 'Qian/Chien', which means Heaven; while in using *Lu* we divert the opponent's arms by placing our hand/s above his and diverting it/them to the side and behind us – that is, towards the trigram 'Kun', which means Earth.

Likewise *Ji*, a straight attack such as a push or palm strike, usually follows *Peng* and is therefore at right angles to *Peng*; while *An*, downward press, is usually employed after *Lu* and was therefore also at right angles to *Lu*. *Cai*, to uproot, is usually used diagonally upwards in an arc; while *Lie*, spiralling force, is usually used diagonally downwards in an arc. *Zhou*, the use of the elbow/forearm, is usually employed diagonally upwards, while *Kao*, to lean/use the shoulder, is used diagonally downwards.

Fig. 68 The relationship of the Five Elements and the Five Steps.

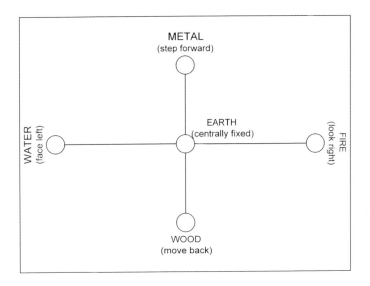

Kao and *Cai* are not methods peculiar to TCC, but appear in the text of the *Classic of Boxing* and are employed in Praying Mantis Boxing.

The Five Steps are linked with the Five Elements because the Five Elements have Yin and Yang qualities and a positive or negative relationship to one another. For example, Metal destroys Wood, and Water extinguishes Fire. Earth is the key element and so occupies the central position; on the one hand it produces Metal and Wood, on the other it can destroy both Fire and Water.

Though the TCC Classics list the Five Elements in the order 'Metal, Wood, Water, Fire and Earth', there were three other major arrangements. For our purposes the most important of these are expressed in the Ho Tu (Yellow River Diagram) and the Lo Shu (Lo River Drawing).

The *Book of Changes* states '...the diagram comes from the Yellow River; the drawing is from the Lo River. The sage from these creates the Eight Trigrams'. This refers to the legendary origins of the two basic arrangements of the Five Elements, the Ho Tu (Yellow River Diagram) being found on

the back of a dragon horse that lived in the Yellow River, while the Lo Shu (Lo River Drawing) was found on the carapace of an immortal tortoise from that river. The first is a clockwise and mutually generative cycle, with each element in turn giving birth to the next; the second is an anti-clockwise and mutually destructive cycle with each element in turn destroying the next.

In the generative cycle:
Metal gives birth to Water
Water gives birth to Wood
Wood gives birth to Fire
Fire gives birth to Earth
Earth gives birth to Metal

In the destructive cycle:
Metal destroys Wood
Wood destroys Earth
Earth destroys Water
Water destroys Fire
Fire destroys Metal

Each element is also held to be stronger than the element that gave birth to it: thus Metal gives birth to Water, so Water is stronger

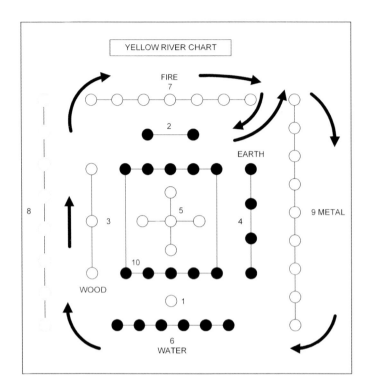

YELLOW RIVER CHART

FIRE
7

2

EARTH

8

5

3

4

9 METAL

10

WOOD

1

6
WATER

Fig. 69 The Five Elements in the generative cycle.

than Metal. When any element is opposed by another quantity of the same element, the stronger element will win.

To sum up, any element is stronger than two of the other four elements and weaker than the other two. The interaction between the elements is eternal and continuous. Each element has both Yin and Yang characteristics. Thus Metal could be sharp and shiny or rusty and dull, while Water could be a roaring waterfall or a muddy pool.

TCC has a self-defence drill called Five Element Arm; despite the name, there is no direct correlation to the references to the Five Elements that appear in this Classic.

Linking the Five Steps and the Five Elements, if we use Metal (advance in a straight line) and the opponent also uses Metal (advances in a straight line), then the stronger force will prevail. It makes more sense to use Fire or Water and evade the attack, or to use Centrally Stable or Move Back in conjunction with a diversion to redirect the opponent to one side or the other.

The Five Steps are of key importance in using TCC as a fighting art. They are trained to some extent in the hand and weapon forms and the Tai Chi Nei Kung, but more so in evasion drills such as *Fu Yang* (Bow Down, Look Up) and *Cai Lang* (the Uprooting Wave). Footwork is often much neglected in TCC. This is partly the fault of Yang Chengfu, who is shown in Yang family books using self-defence applications in a way that might have worked for him with his massive build, but which would be absurd for a small person dealing with a larger opponent.

Centrally Stable is identified with Earth. Earth is the key element, as all the others are found in, on, or under it. Centrally Stable is the position from which the other steps spring, and to which we return. Face Left

Fig. 70 The Five Elements in the destructive cycle.

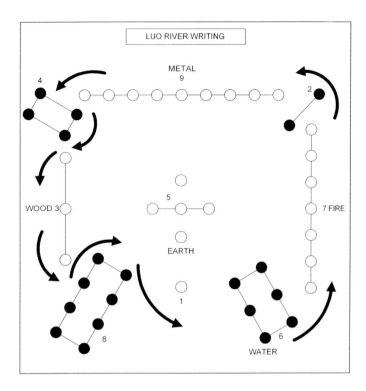

and Look Right take their places as Water and Fire respectively, while Step Forwards is Metal, and Move Back is Wood. TCC makes extensive use of evasion and counterattack, as well as the Chinese military stratagem of retreating in order to advance. Students are often confused by the terms Face Left and Look Right, but they are only a poetic way of telling us to sidestep the opponent's attack while keeping an eye on him.

Here again, the first essay in the series of forty writings published by the Yang and Wu families, and therefore having their presumed endorsement, gives a different relationship between the Five Elements and the Five Steps than that given in the Classics; another likely example of carelessness rather than recondite knowledge (*see* Fig. 68) gives

the normal arrangement of the Five Steps according to Five Element theory.

Centrally Stable is being well balanced or centred and focused. The Great Learning states that only when we are stable can we attain peace and calm. When asked about meditation some years ago, the Dalai Lama stated that without peace of mind it is impossible to meditate; the same thing applies to fighting.

Linking each of the Eight Forces to one of the Eight Trigrams, and each of the Five Steps to one of the Five Elements, is artificial. It helps in analysing TCC techniques; it is not a straitjacket, though this has not stopped some practitioners from using it as such and insisting that everyone else does the same.

8 Classic 2: The Canon of Tai Chi Chuan (*Tai Chi Chuan Ching*)

Some authorities have *Tai Chi Chuan Ching* (the Canon of Tai Chi Chuan) as the title for Classic 1, and *Tai Chi Chuan Lun* for the present text. I have given the titles as I was taught them; the content is more important than the title.

The term '*Ching*' will be familiar to those who are interested in Chinese philosophy. It appears in the titles of works such as '*I Ching*', '*Tao Te Ching*' and many others. It is often translated as 'book' or 'Classic', but here I prefer 'canon', which is derived from a Greek term meaning 'measuring line' or 'standard'. Its primary meaning is a code or regulation made by ecclesiastical authority. The use of this term in the title points to the strong philosophical and cosmological element in this particular text. The text is heavily influenced by Zhou Dun-yi's (AD1017–1073) *Tai Chi Tu Shuo* (Supreme Pole (Tai Chi) Diagram Explanation), which we will examine in Part III.

The present text is often attributed to Wang Zong-yue, a martial artist and scholar active in the late eighteenth century. There are many references to duality, such as movement and stillness, separation and unity, exaggerated and lacking, bent then straight, hard and stiff, pliant and soft, and the TCC approach is contrasted with that of external martial arts.

TCC Classic 2

Tai Chi (the Supreme Ultimate),
It was born from Wu Chi (No Ultimate).
It produces both movement and stillness;
It is the mother of Yin and Yang.
Once there is movement, there is separation.
Once there is stillness, there is unity.
There is nothing exaggerated,
nor is anything lacking.
Sui (follow) bending then straightening,
When the opponent is hard and stiff
and I am pliant and soft, this
is called Zou (moving);
When I am smooth and the opponent is
not, this is called Nian (adherence);
If the opponent's actions are swift,
then my response is swift.
If his actions are slow then I
slowly Sui (follow) them.
Although there are 10,000 transformations,
The principles remain the same.
Through practice and familiarity
(Zhao Shu), we gradually come to
understand Jin (trained force).
From understanding Jin, we can achieve
enlightenment (Shen Ming),
However, we must be diligent
over a long period of time,
And cannot suddenly become expert.

Empty the neck and headtop of strength,
The Qi (vital energy) sinks to the
Dan Tian (region of vital heat).
Don't lean to either side or forwards or back,
Suddenly conceal, suddenly reveal,
When the left feels heavy then
make the left empty,
When the right feels heavy then
make the right distant,
When the opponent looks up, I am still higher;
When he looks down, I am lower still.
When he advances, the
distance seems surpassingly long,
When he retreats, the distance
seems surpassingly short.
A feather cannot be added,
A fly cannot land,
Nobody knows me,
I alone know them,
A hero thus becomes invincible.
Other schools of martial arts are so numerous
Although there are external differences,
Without exception, they amount to nothing
more than the strong bullying the weak;
The slow surrendering to the fast;
The powerful beating those without power;
Slow hands surrendering to fast hands.
This is entirely due to innate (Prior
to Heaven) natural ability
It is not related to having learned the
skilful use of Li (strength) at all.
From the sentence, 'Four taels (Chinese ounce)
displace a thousand catties (Chinese pound).'
It is evident we do not use force
to get the upper hand.
When we observe an old man of eighty
withstanding the assault of a group of people,
How can it be due to speed?
Stand like a level scale,
Move like a wheel.
Sink the weight on one side then Sui (follow),
With double-weightedness then
there is a hindrance.

You can often see people, who have
practised their skills for several years,
But who still cannot change and turn.
This leads to their being entirely
regulated by others.
They are not aware of their
sickness of double-weightedness.
If we wish to be free from this sickness,
We must know Yin and Yang.
When Nian (adherence) is
simply Zou (moving),
When Zou is simply Nian,
When Yin does not depart from Yang,
When Yang does not depart from Yin,
When Yin and Yang aid one another,
Then we can say that we
understand Jin (trained force).
After we understand Jin,
The more we train, the more expert we become.
Silently memorize, study and imitate.
Gradually we reach the point
where we can do all we wish,
Originally it is giving up
yourself to follow the opponent,
Many err by forsaking what is
near to pursue what is far.
It is said, 'A minute discrepancy leads to an
error of one thousand Li (Chinese mile).'
The student must carefully discriminate.

Commentary

Tai Chi,
It was born from Wu Chi.
It produces both movement and stillness;
It is the mother of Yin and Yang.

The term *Chi* means 'limit' or 'ultimate'; Lao Tzu uses it in this sense in the *Tao Te Ching* on a number of occasions. Wu Chi means 'no ultimate'/'without limit', as opposed to Tai Chi, the 'supreme ultimate'. It can be found in a passage of the *Zuo Chuan*, the commentary on the *Spring and Autumn Annals*, written by a disciple of Confucius at the beginning of the third century BC, where women are described as being *Wu Chi* or 'without limit' in their desires. Lao Tzu wrote about returning to a state of *Wu Chi* in the sense of the infinite, which is precisely what happens in Tai Chi hand forms; the final position, like the first position, is often described as Wu Chi. Forms are journeys, like life: a return to where we started.

Lao Tzu said, '...Something and nothing mutually give birth to each other,' (*Tao Te Ching*, Ch. 2). Chuang Tzu wrote that there was a beginning; a beginning before that beginning; and a beginning previous to that beginning before there was a beginning. Tai Chi may have been a later concept, because the first known reference to Tai Chi in Chinese literature is in Appendix III of the *Book of Changes* (*I Ching/Yi Jing*), which dates from around the second century BC. It states:

> The *I* (*Book of Changes*) has Tai Chi (the Great Ultimate),
> It gives birth to the Two Forms (Yin and Yang).

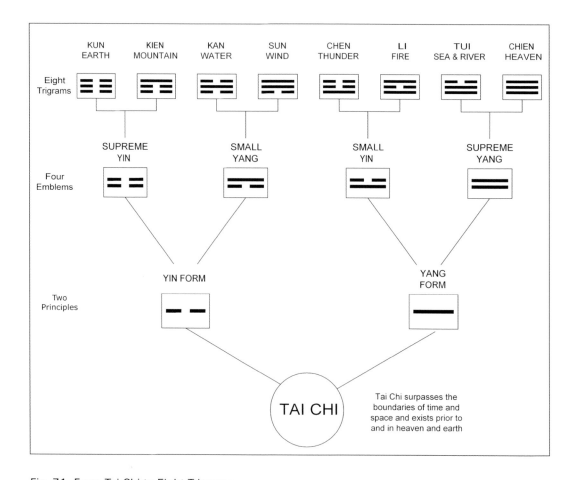

Fig. 71 From Tai Chi to Eight Trigrams.

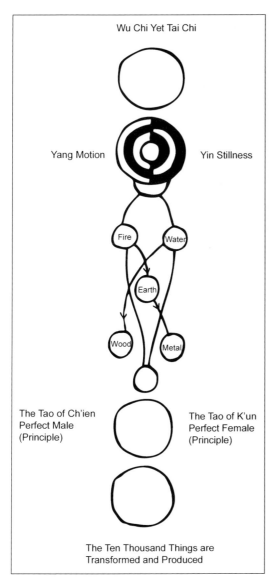

Fig. 72 Tai Chi Diagram of Zhou Dun-yi.

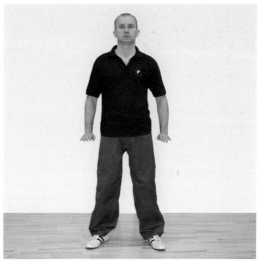

Fig. 73 Tai Chi at Rest or Wu Chi.

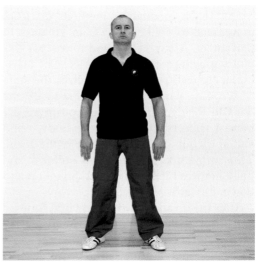

Fig. 74 Tai Chi Ready Position or Tai Chi.

The Two Principles give birth
to the Four Emblems;
The Four Emblems give birth
to the Eight Trigrams.

The first two paragraphs of this Classic are borrowing directly from the *Tai Chi Diagram*

Explanation of Zhou Dun-yi (1017–73). This will be dealt with in Part III.

Once there is movement, there is separation.
Once there is stillness, there is unity.
There is nothing exaggerated,
nor is anything lacking.

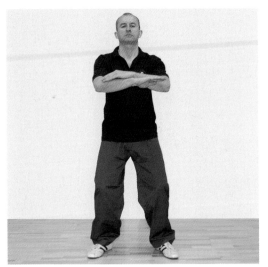

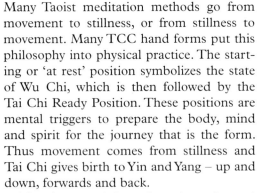

Fig. 75 Tai Chi in Unity/Harmony.

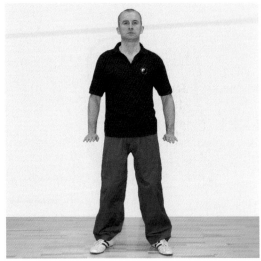

Fig. 76 Wu Chi/Tai Chi at Rest.

Many Taoist meditation methods go from movement to stillness, or from stillness to movement. Many TCC hand forms put this philosophy into physical practice. The starting or 'at rest' position symbolizes the state of Wu Chi, which is then followed by the Tai Chi Ready Position. These positions are mental triggers to prepare the body, mind and spirit for the journey that is the form. Thus movement comes from stillness and Tai Chi gives birth to Yin and Yang – up and down, forwards and back.

After the up and down, in and out, forward and back dualities of the form journey, we arrive at a Tai Chi in Unity/Harmony posture, and conclude with a return to the original Wu Chi/Tai Chi at Rest posture. The stillness referred to is this reuniting of Yin and Yang. 'The female constantly gets the better of the male by stillness,' (*Tao Te Ching* Ch. 61).

This unity or oneness is to be found in the Nei Kung exercise Embracing the One, to which the practitioner returns briefly before moving on to the next technique. It acts as a kind of physical Chinese neurolinguistic programming to prepare mind and body

for what is coming next. Likewise in Yang lineage forms there is a constant return to Seven Stars (also known as Stroke the Lute) to prepare for the next opponent.

Once we have movement, we immediately have a separation of Tai Chi into Yin and Yang. All techniques come from, and contain, Yin and Yang, and Tai Chi is the mother of all this. Separation comes as soon as we commence the form proper; there is front and back, up and down, left and right. The hand form contains specific techniques using the term 'separate', such as 'Separate Hands' and 'Separate Feet'.

'Nothing exaggerated' or 'lacking' requires techniques to be neither too big nor too small, both in forms and in self-defence. If movements are too big, correct alignment is destroyed. In TCC forms competition, many competitors exaggerate their stances and limb extension to impress the judges, but through the same process, damage their joints. Many teachers, when they get older or when teaching the less agile, fail to sink into their stances and root the feet, and fail to contract and extend the limbs sufficiently.

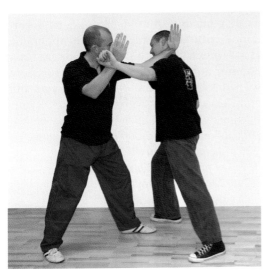

Fig. 77 Separate Arms.

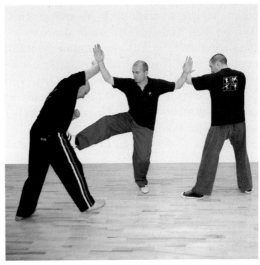

Fig. 78 Separate Feet.

Students who copy such teachers, will get only limited benefits from their practice; the body is not strengthened as much as it could be, and there is limited stimulation of the circulation and respiration.

If defensive movements are exaggerated, they take longer to complete and so our response to an attack is less immediate; if the movements are lacking, we fail to protect a big enough area, or the structure is not sufficient to meet the attack. Likewise, if our counter is too strong and is unsuccessful, we leave ourselves vulnerable to a riposte; if it is lacking, it will lack penetration and will annoy rather than hurt the opponent.

Even when the arms are straight in the sense of focused – for example, at the completion of 'Brush Knee Twist Step' – the joints are rounded (slightly bent) and not locked out to make the striking arm and rear leg perfectly straight. The phrase 'no excess, no deficiency' is also a reference to the small black and white circles found inside the Tai Chi symbol's Yang and Yin aspects respectively. We avoid being 100 per cent Yin or 100 per cent Yang and are thus able to change at any time.

Sui (follow) bending then straightening,
When the opponent is hard and stiff and I am
pliant and soft, this is called Zou (moving);

Sui (follow) is a strategy to respond to an opponent. In TCC practice we constantly bend and straighten the arms, legs and body, both for martial and therapeutic reasons. We will bend the arms to defend against an attack, then straighten them to hit the opponent; the legs and body similarly bend and straighten as we apply force. The opponent's movements may also be bent – that is, twisted or in a curve or maybe a straight line, and we respond accordingly. This is a practical interpretation of Lao Tzu's words: 'Great fullness as if empty; use will not drain it. Great straightness as if bent...' (*Tao Te Ching* Ch. 45).

'*Zou*' means 'to move'/'run'/'go', though in many TCC books it is translated as 'neutralize'. Here it is the strategy of moving in any direction in accordance with the opponent's movements. This can only be achieved by being both pliant and soft instead of becoming hard and stiff like him. If we are stiff, we will be unable to respond to his movements. As Lao Tzu had it, 'The weak overcoming the strong, and the soft overcoming the hard; everyone in the world knows, but no one is able to do it' (*Tao Te Ching* Ch. 78). The *Classic of Boxing* states: 'When you want to be soft, know how to match (the opponent) with oblique evasion.'

Many TCC practitioners over-emphasize softness; as in life, the key is to be soft at the right time and hard at the right time. Softness isn't just a matter for the hands and arms; in many TCC techniques the softness used in defence consists of interception of an attack combined with '...oblique evasion'.

When I am smooth and the opponent is
not, this is called adherence (Nian);
If the opponent's actions are swift,
then my response is swift;

'*Nian*' means 'to adhere'/'stick'. It is the strategy of intercepting, controlling and smoothly redirecting the opponent's force, rather than using force against force by blocking his attack. This is accomplished by total body movement, thus changing the angle and distance. This strategy is also used in other Chinese martial arts, such as Praying Mantis Boxing.

If his actions are slow then I
slowly Sui (follow) them.

I have translated '*Sui*' as 'follow' rather than the more usual translation of 'yield', because the process of '*Sui*' can involve moving in any direction in response to his pressure, and is not just a matter of retreating. A key concept from the Complete Reality/Truth sect of Taoism emphasized *following* nature, in every sense.

Although these concepts are to be applied physically, this is impossible without the proper mental attitude. We should not have a set plan, but should respond in accordance with the changes of the opponent. If we move too soon our opponent may counter our attempted counter; if too slow, we will be hit before we have started our counter.

Although there are 10,000 transformations,
The principles remain the same.
Through practice and familiarity
(Zhao Shu), we gradually come to
understand Jin (trained force).
From understanding Jin, we can achieve
enlightenment (Shen Ming),
However, we must be diligent
over a long period of time,
And cannot suddenly become expert.

Techniques are limitless, but the basic principles of Yin and Yang remain the same. 'Through practice and familiarity...' doesn't give the full flavour of '*Zhao Shu*'. The character for '*Zhao*' has four different possible pronunciations: one of its meanings is 'to play a trick in chess' (Chinese chess requires two players); here it means (through practice) 'to arrive at'. '*Shu*' means 'ripe'/'familiar'/'skilled'. So '*Zhao Shu*' is 'becoming familiar with techniques through practice with others'.

I have rendered '*Shen Ming*' as 'achieve enlightenment'. As in Chan Buddhism: this enlightenment may be gradual or sudden. '*Shen*' is 'spirit' or 'spiritual essence'. The character for '*Ming*' is sun and moon together, thus brightness and illumination, Yin and Yang; this is also the second level in Chinese chess. The whole phrase has the idea of spiritual illumination.

'*Jin*', or 'trained force', can be used in defence or attack; the term also appears in Classics 3 and 5. It is a general concept in Chinese martial arts and not unique to TCC. Internal martial arts use internal force (*Nei Jin*). In defence this involves using a turning or sliding force to intercept, blend with and dissipate the opponent's technique. In counterattacking, it involves a sudden transformation from soft to hard. We can only understand *Jin* through concentrating on total body movement and by training with many different partners in pushing hands and self-defence.

Understanding *Jin* is a three-step process. The first step is '*Ting Jin*'. '*Ting*' literally means 'to listen'/'to hear'. The character for *Ting* consists of the following component characters: disciple, ten, ear(s), eye(s) and heart (mind). So we have a disciple with the greatest concentration (ten times) using the information detected by his senses (eyes and ears) to decide (use mind) what is happening and how to respond to it. Here this means to detect where the opponent's *Jin* is coming from, and where it is going. At a distance from the opponent we can use our eyes to detect this, but when we are at close quarters we should either be hitting the opponent or should have physical contact with his hands or arms so that we can '*Ting*'. Failure to

hit him or to have contact will give him the opportunity to hit us.

The second step is '*Hua Jin*'. '*Hua*' is 'to change'/'transform'/'influence'; here it involves using defensive *Jin*, to redirect the opponent's *Jin* away from him or back into him; to do this we must be relaxed so that we can follow, adhere and move effectively.

The third step is '*Fa Jin*' or to discharge *Jin*, where we use *Jin* to counterattack the opponent. The ability to discharge effectively requires conditioning training, including Tai Chi Nei Kung. This process of *Ting, Hua, Fa* should be instantaneous.

Empty the neck and headtop of strength,
The Qi sinks to the Dan Tian (region of vital heat).
Don't lean to either side or forwards or back,
Suddenly conceal, suddenly reveal,

I have translated '*Xu Ling Ding Jin*' as 'Empty the neck and headtop of strength...': this requires us to relax the neck and align the head correctly. We must avoid rigidity in

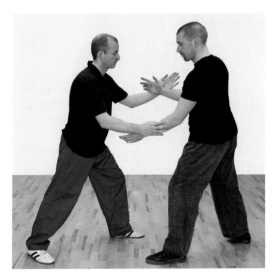

Fig. 79 *Ting* – listening.

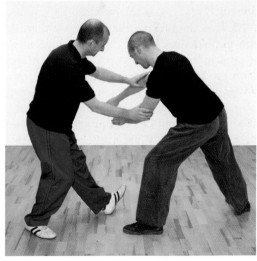

Fig. 80 *Hua* – transform.

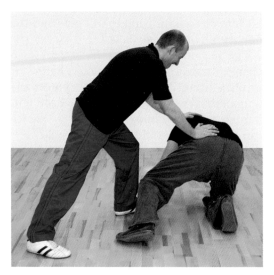

Fig. 81 *Fa* – discharge.

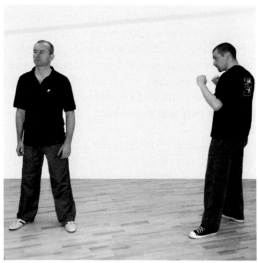

Fig. 82 Opponent prepares to attack from behind and to the side.

the head and neck, otherwise the *Jingshen* (a combination of essence and spirit, and meaning vigour) is affected and so balance is clumsy; correct alignment makes head and neck empty, and being empty, they go with the *Jin*. However, in self-defence, inclining the head to one side makes it easier to use body evasion or a sidestep to avoid an attack.

Another important reason for not twisting the head and neck out of alignment in normal practice, and instead moving them with the torso, is to train peripheral vision, an important quality in any martial artist. Normally when people turn round, they turn the head first, but in TCC practice, the head turns with the body and not separately. Continuous practice will develop the peripheral vision – seeing without looking.

That *Qi* (vital energy) sinks to the *Dan Tian* (region of vital heat) is a poetic reference implying deep abdominal breathing. This breathing helps us to drop the centre of gravity and root our feet in the ground so that we don't become top heavy. All breathing is done through the nose, so that air is

filtered by the mucous membranes and warmed before it goes into the lungs. By developing relaxation through slow practice of form and Tai Chi Nei Kung, the lungs are

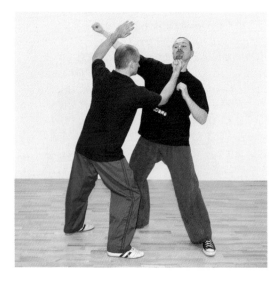

Fig. 83 Defender detects the attack using peripheral vision and responds with Turn around Swing Fist.

able to expand further down than normal. This process can be seen and felt at the area of the *Dan Tian*. Ironically this is bad news for smokers, because they are able to inhale more effectively.

Normally we will fight from a neutral position, not leaning to either side, and only inclining when it is necessary to avoid or to hit an opponent. Aligning the head properly is essential for balance – hence the statement that we shouldn't lean. It also aids the effective functioning of the nervous system and keeps open the airways so we can take an optimal amount of oxygen into the lungs, allowing them to extend downwards and produce the effect referred to as 'sinking the *Qi* to the *Dan Tian*'.

There are three '*Dan Tian*': the first is between the eyebrows, the second is just below the level of the heart, and the third (the one referred to here) is a point about two inches below the navel. Each region is said to consist of nine cavities.

Dan Tian is often translated literally as 'cinnabar field', and is also referred to as the 'sea of breath'. A better translation, used by Professor Joseph Needham, is 'region of vital heat', a reference to one of the theoretical staging posts in the creation of an 'inner elixir' or *Nei Dan* by the use of respiratory techniques. In Taoist theory, attainment of this inner elixir leads to the state referred to as 'long life, not old': that is, longevity without the infirmities of age. This is one of the reasons for TCC's popularity with the literati. However, I don't yet know of any immortals created by this process.

In a discussion at the Tai Chi Caledonia event some years back, All China champion, Wang Hai-jun, said that when pushing hands he would first sink his *Qi* to the *Dan Tian*: in Western terms this meant he would be immediately centred and focused. For our purposes, the *Qi* sinking to the *Dan Tian* means that, when practising the form, the

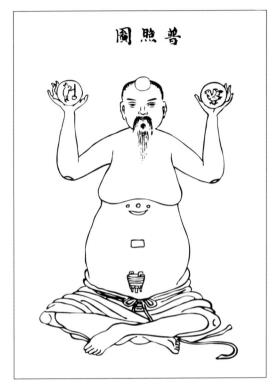

Fig. 84 The three *Dan Tian*. Note the rabbit pounding the mortar in the right hand – a metaphor for Internal Alchemy also referred to in the Tai Chi Nei Kung technique, Jade Rabbit faces Moon.

relaxed state produced promotes abdominal breathing, and we can see and feel the abdomen contract and expand in tune with the respiration. In addition as we constantly swallow saliva when doing the form, air is brought down into the stomach, and this can cause a degree of flatulence. This is not something to worry about, but can be socially embarrassing. Lao Tzu refers to this abdominal breathing, which is used by babies, when he asks, 'In concentrating your *Qi*, can you become soft as a baby?' (*Tao Te Ching*, Ch.10).

The admonition to avoid leaning is often misunderstood. What we must avoid is leaning

73

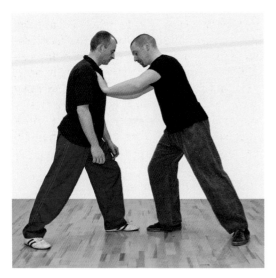

Fig. 85 Opponent pushes.

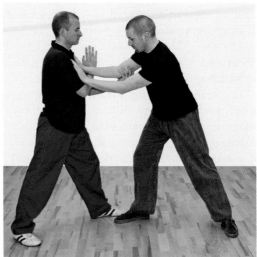

Fig. 86 Turn and divert the push.

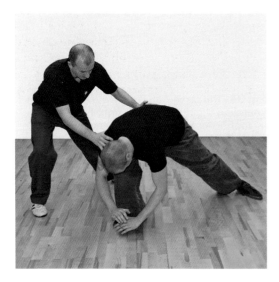

Fig. 87 Opponent is led off-balance into the void.

the head in any direction out of alignment with the neck; this is to keep the alignment from the crown of the head to the tailbone, which strengthens the spine and also aligns the central nervous system running through it to the brain, producing a tranquil state of mind. It is, however, wrong to keep stiffly erect at all times, and indeed in most TCC styles there are movements requiring us to lean the body in one direction or another. If you're not sure, look at photos of famous masters such as Sun Lu-tang, Wu Jian-quan and Yang Cheng-fu.

The practice of not leaning the head to one side or the other is, however, only to be observed when we are training Tai Chi Nei Kung or form, or when we are refining a technique in two-person drills. In free wrestling, or in fighting with or without weapons, it is not only permissible, but advisable to move the head independently, most especially when it is the opponent's first target.

In 1982, I was attacked one afternoon in Nathan Road, Hong Kong. I felt, or maybe with peripheral vision noticed something wrong, and moved my head to one side: a fist came whizzing past from behind – and missed. A fight started, and I didn't feel I'd broken any golden rule from the Classics.

'Suddenly conceal, suddenly reveal': again the emphasis is on bewildering the opponent with change and duality; switching back and forth between hard and soft, straight and circular, the feint and the genuine technique.

When the left feels heavy then
make the left empty
When the right feels heavy then
make the right distant,
When the opponent looks up, I am still higher;
When he looks down, I am lower still.
When he advances, the distance
seems surpassingly long,
When he retreats, the distance
seems surpassingly short.

This paraphrases Lao Tzu, who wrote, 'Long and short offset each other. High and the low incline towards each other… Before and after follow each other' (*Tao Te Ching* Ch. 2). And 'Heavy is the root of light; still is the lord of restless' (*Tao Te Ching* Ch. 26).

TCC is mainly a counterattacking style, where we conceal our intention (or seem still) until the moment of the opponent's attack, when it is revealed in our response. When he puts pressure on, or attacks us in one direction, rather than resisting, we confront him with emptiness by either diverting his force away from us or by removing ourselves from the path of his force, and then counterattack as he is unbalanced.

Being still higher or lower than the opponent means that if his force is directed upwards, we direct it even further upwards; likewise, if it is directed downwards, we direct it yet further down, rather than resisting. This is an example of using Yin to overcome Yang. I have been kicked at many times, and my normal response is to sidestep and scoop upwards, adding to the oncoming force: this technique is called 'Single Hand Seize Leg', and most kickers don't get up too quickly when they've been flipped.

By timing our movements exactly in accordance with his we make it impossible for him to close the gap with us when he attacks, thus making the distance seem 'surpassingly long'; but our counterattack follows so quickly that he is unable to withdraw in time, thus making the distance seem 'surpassingly short'. In Chinese military strategy this is 'retreat in order to advance'. Once the opponent's sting has been drawn he is vulnerable to a counterattack.

A feather cannot be added,
A fly cannot land,
Nobody knows me,
I alone know them,
A hero thus becomes invincible.

We should be so alert and relaxed that we are responsive to the slightest change, while making no unnecessary move ourselves. Thus the opponent finds it difficult to fathom our strategy because we are always responding to, or pre-empting his attacks. There are a number of parallel passages in Chinese military strategy and philosophy.

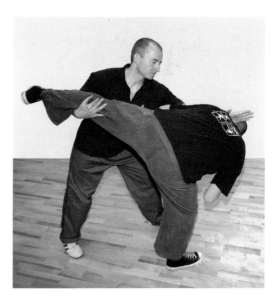

Fig. 88 Single Hand Seize Leg.

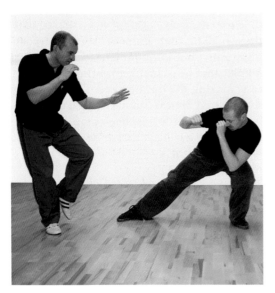

Fig. 89 Stepping back to avoid a sweep.

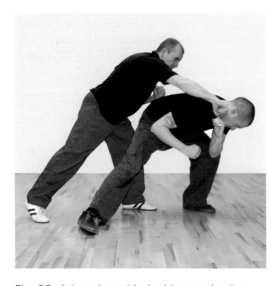

Fig. 90 Advancing with the hit to make the distance surpassingly short.

Sun Tzu said, '…Know the enemy and know yourself, one hundred battles, one hundred victories.' He went on to say that if you do not know the enemy but know yourself, you will sometimes win, sometimes not, but if you know neither yourself nor the enemy you will always be defeated.

As Lao Tzu put it, 'In ancient times, he who acted in accord with the way was minutely subtle, mysteriously comprehending and so profound no one could know him…' (*Tao Te Ching* Ch. 15). And, 'He who knows others is intelligent. He who knows himself is enlightened. He who overcomes others has strength. He who overcomes himself is powerful…' (*Tao Te Ching* Ch. 33). We need to be realistic about our own capacity, and should have knowledge of various styles of fighting so that we can draw conclusions from the posture and guard of an opponent and predict likely attacks.

Other schools of martial arts are so numerous
Although there are external differences,
Without exception, they amount to nothing
more than the strong bullying the weak;
The slow surrendering to the fast;
The powerful beating those without power;
Slow hands surrendering to fast hands.
This is entirely due to innate (prior
to Heaven) natural ability
It is not related to having learned the
skilful use of Li (strength) at all.

This extract is talking about the difference in approach between external martial arts and TCC. Many TCC exponents are deservedly the butt of jokes in the martial arts world, as their arrogance seems to increase in inverse proportion to their fighting abilities. Strength is necessary, but trained strength, not brute strength, for TCC techniques to be effective.

From the sentence, 'Four taels (Chinese ounce)
displace a thousand catties (Chinese pound).'
It is evident we do not use force
to get the upper hand.

When we observe an old man of eighty
withstanding the assault of a group of people,
How can it be due to speed?

Using 'four taels to displace a thousand catties' is a key TCC concept, which we will meet again in Classic 5, and is often misunderstood. We can only accomplish it if, instead of blocking an attack, we use body evasion or footwork, then intercept, add to, and slightly redirect the force with a smooth diversion; this is using Yin to overcome Yang.

TCC pushing hands drills are designed to improve our ability to use the opponent's force against him, to unbalance him and make him vulnerable to our counters, as with Deflect, Parry Punch, lower level. The remark about an old man of eighty is poetic licence, and implies that an older person can defeat a youth, or a lighter person a heavier one, only if the former is well trained. At the time of writing, an old friend, Aidan Cochrane from Belfast, phoned me to say that he'd been in a nightclub fight with three young hoods and

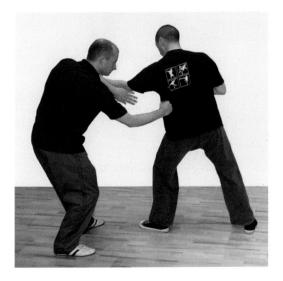

Fig. 91 Deflect, Parry Punch, lower level.

had got hurt, but managed to finish the fight with a Step Back Repulse Monkey on the main guy. That is what the writer is talking about here.

Stand like a level scale,
Move like a wheel.
Sink the weight on one side then Sui (follow),
With double-weightedness then
there is a hindrance.
You can often see people, who have
practised their skills for several years,
But who still cannot change and turn.
This leads to their being entirely
regulated by others.
They are not aware of their
sickness of double-weightedness.
If we wish to be free from this sickness,
We must know Yin and Yang.

Be ready with the shoulders level to move smoothly in response to any pressure, using the concept of rotating the centre line – the spinal column – like a wheel. This rotation of the spinal column is fundamental not only to martial arts, but also to sports as diverse as tennis, golf and discus.

Weight distribution is of fundamental importance and, normally, one foot will be full of weight or rooted, and the other empty; so if wrestling with an opponent we would normally follow his force by using a pull-push circular force action rather than force against force, something that uses a great deal of energy.

Double-weightedness is often misinterpreted as having an even amount of weight on each foot. Every martial art has some movements where the weight is evenly distributed – in every TCC style I can think of, forms start and finish with the feet positioned a shoulder's width apart and the weight evenly distributed. The last line in this section gives the best definition of double-weightedness:

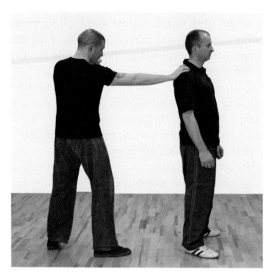

Fig. 92 Opponent makes contact from behind and is ready to punch.

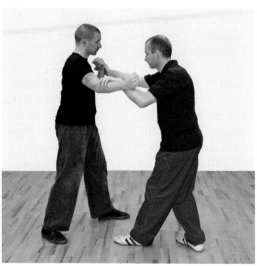

Fig. 93 Turn and fold over his arms.

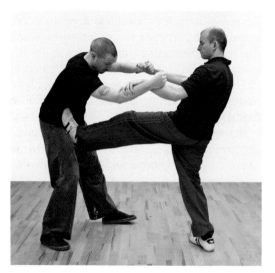

Fig. 94 Once he is trapped, kick with heel.

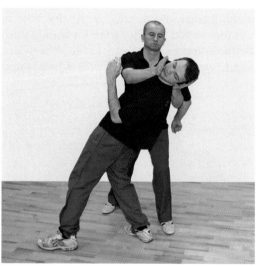

Fig. 95 Pat the Horse High – Ho Chi-minh style, using pull-push circular force.

an absence of Yin and Yang. This arises when we are either unbalanced or tense and so cannot move easily – a sickness. There are more misconceptions here. Even some experienced TCC practitioners teach that one must never move a foot when it is full of weight, but empty it, then move it. However, this is a suicidal approach to fighting.

I would refer such gallants to Jack Dempsey's book *Championship Fighting*, in which he teaches the 'Drop Step'. This involves stepping in with the front foot to jab with the front hand, and is especially devastating when the opponent is coming forwards on to it. I was taught the same technique as a karate beginner in the early 1970s. My son learned to do basically the same thing lungeing with his épée, when he started fencing at the age of six. It is suicidal to shift the weight back before stepping in with the front foot because this telegraphs your intended technique to the opponent, as well as increasing the amount of time it takes to do a technique. Yet this is precisely what many experienced teachers are saying.

Some years ago I was menaced by three young guys after midnight and near my home. The biggest asked what I was looking at. He pulled his fist and weight back, so I hit him once using a drop step. He was unconscious before he hit the ground. In my own form sometimes the one foot is both full and empty. The ball of the foot can be lifted from the ground to reduce friction and allow the foot to turn in or out with the weight still forward on that foot. Sometimes it is smarter to shift weight, but it depends on the technique. It's all a matter of good tuition, practice and common sense.

As for people who have practised their skills for years being unable to turn and change and being regulated by others, this is another reference to the final product: the use of trained skill in a self-defence situation. After acquiring basic evasion, interception, diversion, throwing, locking and striking skills, each application should be practised regularly at speed against an opponent who sometimes attacks on the left, sometimes on the right. There should be a degree of spontaneity in the training, rather than just going through pre-set routines and drills.

Pulls, punches and locks should be applied with torque, a key method taught to karate beginners (though they don't know it, and even if they did, wouldn't know why). Chen TCC people are always talking about silk-reeling, coiling and uncoiling, but in the end it is just torque, or turning and changing.

The weight doesn't have to be predominantly on one leg or the other at all times, but we should be able to move easily at any instant in response to the movements of the opponent. If we know Yin and Yang we can easily effect this change.

When Nian (adherence) is
simply Zou (moving),
When Zou (moving) is simply
Nian (adherence),
When Yin does not depart from Yang,
When Yang does not depart from Yin,
When Yin and Yang aid one another,
Then we can say that we
understand Jin (trained force).

The strategy of Adherence (*Nian*) requires that at close quarters we must have arm contact with the opponent so we can feel what he is doing and counteract it by redirecting his force. The strategy of Moving (*Zou*) means we move the feet or body forwards, back or sideways in response to the movements of the opponent, rather than resisting them. It is not enough to have only *Nian* or only *Zou*; they go together like Yin and Yang. The key is to be or use Yin at the right time, and to be or use Yang at the right time, and to change as required. Chuang Tzu said one should not follow and honour the Yin and ignore the Yang. The overemphasis of Yin is the great weakness of so many TCC practitioners.

After we understand Jin
The more we train, the more
expert we become.

Silently memorize, study and imitate.
Gradually we reach the point
where we can do all we wish,
Originally it is giving up
yourself to follow the opponent,
Many err by forsaking what is
near to pursue what is far.
It is said, 'A minute discrepancy leads to an
error of one thousand Li (Chinese mile).'
The student must carefully discriminate.

I discussed earlier the three-step process involved in understanding force. *Jin* can be hard or soft, Yin or Yang, long or short. 'The more we train, the more expert (*Jing*)...': this *Jing* is the same character that means 'vital essence' in Internal Alchemy. Here it means 'expert', and it is given the same meaning when used to refer to the basic level of mastery in Chinese chess.

'Silently memorize, study and imitate': don't just talk about it, do it! But even this is not enough: it is necessary to ask questions when in doubt, something which many students are strangely reluctant to do.

'....Giving up yourself...' means that rather than having preset notions or plans, we should act in accordance with what the opponent actually does, rather than what we expect him to do, so we must detect and immediately respond to his every change. 'Forsaking what is near to pursue what is far' is where, rather than using a quick and simple diversion, we attempt something overcomplicated, or when counterattacking, pick a target that is out of reach rather than what is nearest to hand.

Small mistakes lead to big mistakes, especially where the person making them is himself a teacher, so it is important to pay attention to every detail. It is more difficult to correct experienced people who have long trained mistakes and bad habits, than to teach a beginner from scratch.

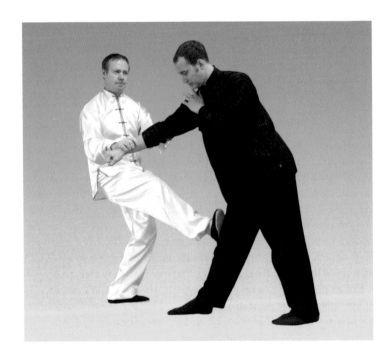

Author demonstrates
a Repulse Monkey
Application.

9 Classic 3: Interpretation of the Practice of the Thirteen Tactics (*Shi San Shi Xing Gong Xin Jie*)

Xin Jie is 'interpretation'/'explanation', something many Chinese concepts require before they can be understood. I've translated '*Shi San Shi*' as Thirteen Tactics rather than Thirteen Movements/Postures, because every technique in the form is supposed to be derived from a combination of one of the Five Steps and the Eight Forces, so their possible permutations are much more varied than would appear from the latter translation. Here *Kung*/*Gong* (these are different romanizations of the same character as in *Kung Fu* and *Qi Gong*) means 'practice' or 'training'.

Sometimes attributed to Yang Lu-chan's student Wu Yu-xiang, this text discusses the actual practice of TCC and the Thirteen Tactics, not just the theory. (Some claim that the 'Thirteen Tactics' is an old name for what we now call Tai Chi Chuan; however, I suspect it was more likely a name given by someone who used the concepts of the Eight Trigrams and Five Elements to analyse an existing art – not every technique fits easily into the Thirteen Tactics.) Strangely, the Thirteen Tactics are not themselves mentioned in the text except in the title. However, they are dealt with individually elsewhere. This classic is concerned with *Qi* more than anything else, and there are no fewer than a dozen references to this concept. The text shows strong influences from Complete Reality School texts such as the *Book of Balance and Harmony*.

TCC Classic 3

Use the Xin (mind) to move
the Qi (vital energy)
Try to let it sink in an orderly manner,
Then it can accumulate and enter the bones.
Use the Qi to move the body;
Try to let it flow without hindrance,
Then we can conveniently act in
accordance with the Xin.
If the Jingshen (vigour) can be raised,
Then there is no need to worry about
leaning the weight to one side.
This is what is meant by the suspended headtop.
The Yi (intent) and the Qi must
be able to interact nimbly
So there is a delightful roundness and liveliness.
This is what is meant by the changes
of void and substantial.
When attacking you must sink
and be completely relaxed,
Concentrating on one direction.
When standing the body should be Zhong
Zheng (centrally straight/correct) and at ease,
To deal with attacks from the eight directions.
Move the Qi as through a pearl
with nine crooked paths.

It goes smoothly everywhere.
Transport the Jin (trained force) like
a hundred times refined steel,
What firmness can it not break?
The appearance is like a hawk seizing a hare;
The Shen (spirit) is like a cat catching a rat.
Be still as a lofty mountain;
Move like a mighty river.
Accumulate the Jin as if drawing a bow;
Fa (discharge) the Jin as if releasing an arrow.
Seek the straight amidst the bent;
Accumulate then discharge.
The Li (strength) comes from the spine;
The steps follow the changes of the body.
To receive is to release,
If contact is broken, then resume the connection.
Moving back and forth there must
be turning over and folding up.
In advancing and retreating there
must be turning and change.
Ultimate softness then becomes
the hardest and firmest.
From the ability to inhale and exhale properly
comes the ability to be nimble and flexible.
By constantly developing the Qi there is no evil.
By using the curve to gather the Jin
there is more than a sufficiency.
The Xin (mind) acts as the commander;
The Qi acts as the flag;
The waist acts as the banner.
First seek to expand (open), then
seek to be compact (close).
Thus you reach fine work neatly done.
It is also said:
First in the Xin (mind), then in the body.
The abdomen is spongy; the Qi is
hoarded to enter the bones;
The Shen (spirit) is at ease
and the body is tranquil.
This must be deeply engraved on the Xin.
Always remember, once there is movement,
there is nothing that does not move.
Once there is stillness there is
nothing that is not still.
When moving back and forth,

The Qi sticks to the back,
It amasses and enters the spine.
Internally it strengthens the Jingshen (vigour);
Externally one exhibits peaceful ease.
Move the way a cat walks.
Mobilize the Jin as if reeling silk from a cocoon.
The body and the Yi (intent) are entirely
concentrated on the Jingshen (vigour),
Not on the Qi.
If on the Qi,
Then there is stagnation.
If there is Qi then there is no Li (strength).
If there is no Qi then there is great strength.
The Qi is like the wheel of a chariot;
The waist is like the axle.

Commentary

Use the Xin (mind) to move
the Qi (vital energy)
Try to let it sink in an orderly manner,
Then it can accumulate and enter the bones.
Use the Qi to move the body;
Try to let it flow without hindrance,
Then we can conveniently act in
accordance with the Xin.

This extract is talking about the *Qi Gong* and Internal Alchemy aspect of TCC; similar wording is used in many non-TCC methods of *Qi Gong* and meditation. The text is *not* telling us to use the mind to direct *Qi* to different parts of the body. For breathing to work properly we need to concentrate the mind on performing slow, smooth and relaxed movements. Thus when practising Yin aspects of TCC such as the hand form, the internal organs also become relaxed and more flexible, allowing the diaphragm to extend further down than normal when we inhale. This allows the lungs to extend further down, enabling us to take in more oxygen. The increased lung capacity causes the circulation to be stronger than normal.

In Classic 2, this simple physical process is referred to as sinking the *Qi* to the *Dan Tian* (Cinnabar Field).

When practising TCC, we inhale and exhale through the nose with the tip of the tongue pressing against the front of the palate so that we can salivate and thus lubricate the throat. Breathing through the nose filters impurities from the air (*Qi*) and helps to heat it before it reaches the lungs. It is usual to breathe out when the limbs are extended, and in when they are retracted, but many TCC movements are more complex than this. Breathing is deep when we inhale and long when we exhale, so that a maximum amount of *Qi*/oxygen is taken into the lungs, and a maximum amount is absorbed into the bloodstream to pass nutrients to the body and remove waste products, before being exhaled in the form of carbon dioxide (or methane gas).

For *Qi* to accumulate, slow practice of both form and certain Tai Chi Nei Kung exercises is essential. Many people concentrate on breathing in esoteric ways, and end up with poor quality technique. It is the body movements and postures that manipulate the respiration, circulation and central nervous system. There is plenty for the mind to concentrate on – posture, stance, relaxation, co-ordination, the various dualities of opening and closing, rising and sinking, full and empty. Correct practice leads to correct breathing. The better our respiration and circulation, the better the body can function; we don't have to think about the breath and can move freely, concentrating on the techniques, whether in self-defence or in form practice. Harmonious movement leads to harmonious breathing.

Qi is not a scientific term, but whatever we call it, studies have shown that TCC practice can help maintain or at least limit reduction in the level of bone mass density in, for example, post-menopausal women.

The elderly often suffer badly from falls due to problems with balance, posture, flexibility and co-ordination, and the bones are more brittle because of disuse. All these problems can be addressed by regular practice of the more *Yin* aspects of TCC.

If the Jingshen (vigour) can be raised,
Then there is no need to worry about
leaning the weight to one side.
This is what is meant by the suspended headtop.

This term '*Jingshen*' is interesting; most translations of the Classics translate it as 'spirit' and leave it at that, but there is more to it. Taoists have three primary vitalities or treasures, which all life possesses at birth. Primary *Jing*, or seed, becomes the semen or vaginal secretions. Primary *Qi* or 'vital energy' becomes the *Qi* of respiration and circulation. Lastly, primary *Shen* or 'spirit' becomes mental and intellectual activity. This transformation of each of the three primary vitalities could weaken the body, so the Chinese developed ways to increase the level of these vitalities.

'*Jingshen*', literally seed and spirit, is better translated as vigour, both mental and physical. It can be raised by exercise, effective respiration and good posture. This is where 'suspended headtop' is important.

Suspended headtop is an oft-misunderstood concept. Certain zealots would have the crown of the head positioned at all times as if directly suspended from the ceiling, regardless of the technique being performed. This extract is only saying that the head should be correctly aligned with the spine, so that neither it nor the body leans unnecessarily in any direction, thus adversely affecting the balance. In addition the central nervous system functions better with good posture.

The ceiling is only a concept; in actuality the 'ceiling' changes position so that it maintains its relationship to the crown of the head

83

and the coccyx. It is both uncomfortable and absurd to take all this literally and force the headtop and spine to be as if suspended from an actual ceiling at all times. Certain postures are exactly erect, others are not, but in the majority of postures there should be this fairly straight line from the crown of the head to the tailbone. However, the human body has certain natural contours, and should never be stiff like a board. Furthermore, in a self-defence situation, or even when practising free pushing hands, trying to maintain a suspended headtop at all times is ridiculous as well as inappropriate.

The Yi (intent) and the Qi must
be able to interact nimbly
So there is a delightful roundness and liveliness.
This is what is meant by the changes
of void and substantial.

Intent dictates where the techniques go, and the techniques regulate the breath; if intent is absent there is hesitancy or tension and the breath is adversely affected. 'Substantial' means 'full' or 'extended' while 'void' is 'empty' or 'contracted'. 'Substantial' is Yin in that it is dead energy, having reached its extreme, while 'void' is latent energy and so Yang. This is why terms such as 'nimble', 'round' and 'lively' appear in the text; it is the opposite of being stiff and jerky. This goes hand in hand with a tranquil mind.

When practising TCC, normally one foot is substantial (full) and therefore has almost all the weight on it, while the other foot is void (empty) and therefore has very little weight on it – although the one foot can be partly full and partly empty as when we wish to turn round without shifting the weight completely back first. We should also constantly extend and contract the torso, the arms and legs and the hands and fingers.

Constant weight transference, coupled with contracting and expansive movements,

make the circulation stronger. With concentration on these points and good respiration we will feel smooth and lively and be able to effect changes of substantial and void with ease. There is a similar full and empty with regard to the air (*Qi*) in the lungs and, as with the limbs, we don't completely fill or empty the lungs. This is what is meant by the effective interaction of *Yi* and *Qi*. Everything is controlled and harmonious.

When attacking you must sink
and be completely relaxed,
Concentrating on one direction.
When standing the body should be Zhong
Zheng (centrally straight/correct) and at ease,
To deal with attacks from the eight directions.

So that we can move with maximum speed when attacking an opponent, we must be relaxed and rooted, then we can change and move easily from one position to another. Rooting is done by lowering the centre of gravity – that is, sinking. Formerly this was referred to as moving from one trigram to another; this usage is now obsolete, though a vestige of it remains in moving step pushing hands drills such as Eight Gates, Five Steps and Nine Palace Step. The centre line of the body, and therefore the bodyweight, should be going in the direction of any technique we apply, otherwise we are only using the strength of the limbs.

Concentrating in one direction requires that when thrusting forwards, as in Tai Chi Spear, the spear point, the nose and front knee all point in the direction of the thrust (*see* Fig. 96 overleaf).

Zhong Zheng (centrally straight/correct) is talking about correct, but relaxed alignment of the crown of the head, spinal column and coccyx. TCC Classic 4 explains how to be *Zhong Zheng* through correct body alignment. 'At ease' is to neither hunch forwards nor bend back as we await the opponent's

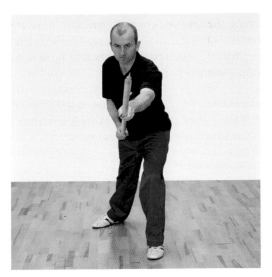

Fig. 96 Following the spear three-tip rule.

also be talking about the nine major sections of the body (head, neck, shoulder, elbow, wrist, waist, hip, knee and ankle), all connected ultimately to the spine and therefore the central nervous system. The *Qi* is constantly being threaded in all nine of them, which are all crooked when they are in motion.

More simply, the blood flows to and from the heart through a complex network of veins and arteries. Slow movement, combined with raising and lowering, contracting and expanding, coiling and uncoiling, closing and opening, and so on, stimulates this flow.

Transport the Jin (trained force) like
a hundred times refined steel,
What firmness can it not break?

Jin is compared to refined steel and should therefore be both elastic and resilient. 'A hundred times refined steel' is only made with considerable effort; just so, skill and ability take time and effort to train. Certain Taoist practices require a disciple to train intensively for 100 days; this is directly mentioned in the *Jade Emperor Mind Seal Classic*. In Chinese martial arts this 100-day practice also exists; in Tai Chi Nei Kung training, disciples traditionally practice the twelve *Yin* exercises for 100 days, during which time they refrain from sexual activity. The master then tests the disciple in various ways, such as getting a fellow disciple to jump on his abdomen from shoulder height.

Breaking firmness requires *Jin* to be sudden and concentrated on one specific part of the opponent's body. Like many other martial arts, TCC has sudden and sharp use of *Jin*; this is trained in both Tai Chi Nei Kung and some ancillary training methods.

attack. We should always be ready to change from attack to defence against attacks from any direction, as with the concept of being centrally fixed or with central equilibrium, as we met in Classic 1.

Move the Qi as through a pearl
with nine crooked paths.
It goes smoothly everywhere.

The reference to a pearl is peculiarly Taoist and occurs many times in Li Daoqun's thirteenth-century compilation, the *Book of Balance & Harmony*, with reference to Internal Alchemy. Li also refers to combining nine massage strokes for each exhalation. Each *Dan Tian* is said to consist of nine cavities, and this may be what the author was indirectly alluding to – that is, the *Qi* should permeate the whole body. Alternatively, the text could be referring to the Yellow Emperor's *Canon of Internal Medicine* (compiled around the second century BC), which talks of the nine orifices, all of which require efficient circulation if they are to function properly. The text could

The appearance is like a hawk seizing a hare;
The spirit (Shen) is like a cat catching a rat.

Although relaxed, both hawk and cat have total concentration when hunting and do not make any excessive movements; both are swift and sudden when they pounce on their prey.

Be still as a lofty mountain;
Move like a mighty river.

'Still as a lofty mountain' requires that we should be rooted and balanced at all times. The static exercises in Tai Chi Nei Kung train this. 'Move like a mighty river' requires that our movements should be continuous and flowing, sweeping all before us. Note well that a river changes its speed according to the terrain, and it is just so in a TCC form: though the movements are flowing, they are not all done at the same speed.

Lao Tzu said, 'Under heaven, there is nothing softer and weaker than water, but nothing is more capable in attacking the hard and strong' (*Tao Te Ching* Ch. 78).

TCC makes extensive use of wave-like motion, either in defence or counter-

attack. There is even a specific pushing hands method called *Cai Lang* (the Uprooting Wave), which trains this skill to uproot an opponent.

Accumulate the Jin as if drawing a bow;
Fa (discharge) the Jin as if releasing an arrow.
Seek the straight amidst the bent;
Accumulate then discharge.

Usually TCC defensive movements give us the power for our counterattack. In a technique such as 'Draw Bow to Shoot Tiger' we turn the body in one direction to avoid and divert the opponent's attack; this is to accumulate or to draw the bow. The body turns back in the other direction to discharge the accumulated *Jin* in the form of a double punch to the opponent's face and body; this is discharging as if releasing an arrow. This process can be compared to a coiled spring (accumulate), which is then released (discharge). Many practitioners make too much of '*Fa Jin*': it means to use focused power on an opponent and is

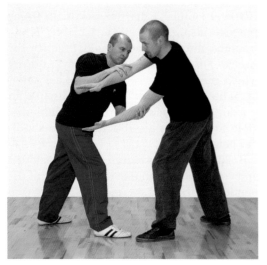 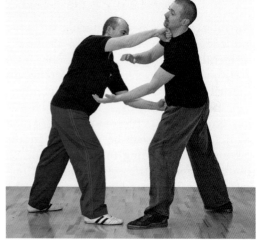

Figs 97 and 98 Draw Bow to Shoot Tiger.

common to all martial arts, though methods vary.

Even when using what appears to be a straight line in TCC, there remains a degree of bend in the striking arm or leg. This represents the Yang in the Yin or the Yin in the Yang, depending whether the technique is defensive or counterattacking. Fully locking the joint damages it, and also makes it more difficult for us to change what we are doing or to follow up our initial response to the opponent's attack. Lao Tzu wrote, '... bent then straight, hollow then full...' (*Tao Te Ching* Ch. 22), so the essence is again in the changes between bent and straight and hollow and full.

The Li (strength) comes from the spine;
The steps follow the changes of the body.
To receive is to release,
If contact is broken then resume the connection.

The spine is the exact centre line of the body; when we exert force we use the centre line – the spine – so that the whole body is doing the technique and not just the arms. If the body needs to move in any direction the weight shifts in that direction, and the feet or at least the stance should shift in the same direction. So when pushing, if we don't actually step forwards, we should at least shift the weight forwards in our stance.

'To receive is to release' means that defending against (receiving) the opponent's attack and counterattacking him (releasing) are not two separate events, but one should follow the other without interruption, to prevent the opponent recovering.

When in contact with the opponent we can control his movements. If contact is broken, we are in imminent danger of being attacked again, so it is imperative that either we hit the opponent first or in some other way regain contact (usually with his arms), so that we can control him, prevent him from hitting us, and use his arms as levers to destroy his balance.

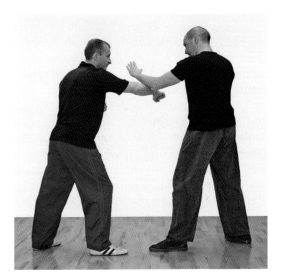 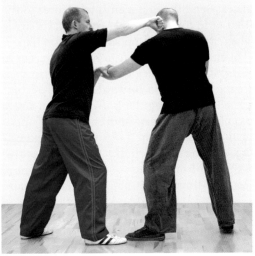

Figs 99 and 100 Gyrating Arms. The punch is blocked, so the puncher follows the direction of the block round in a circle and returns the force of the block with another punch.

*Moving back and forth there must
be turning over and folding up.
In advancing and retreating there
must be turning and change.
Ultimate softness then becomes
the hardest and firmest.*

Turning over and folding up is a key method used by TCC exponents: transition. This transition can be from defence (moving back) to counterattack (moving forwards) where the arms bend and turn to divert and, in a continuous movement in harmony with the steps and body movement, change from soft to hard in order to counterattack. The transition can also be from attack to defence or to another attack. This would be appropriate where the opponent has blocked or countered our response to his initial attack. We soften and go (turning the arm and folding it over) with his force in a wave-like motion, changing to hard again to counter him. The ability to do this is largely trained in 'Gyrating Arms', the core skill in Reeling Silk pushing hands.

We can also, whether in defence or counterattack, bend the opponent's torso over to the front or to the rear, or fold over his arm or leg when, for example, applying a lock on him.

In changing from soft to hard, from Yin to Yang, it is necessary to turn and change as we move back and forwards. This is accomplished by turning the body. There is also a requirement to turn and change the opponent so that he is in a position of disadvantage, setting up a counterattacking opportunity. Also from being soft it is easy to move fast and thus make the application of hard force more powerful. Again, the *Book of Balance and Harmony (Zhong He Ji)* refers to alternating between being firm and yielding and between movement and stillness.

*From the ability to inhale and exhale properly
comes the ability to be nimble and flexible.*

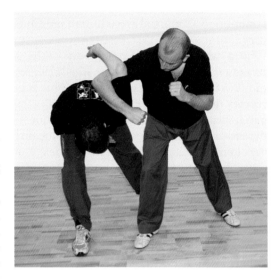

Fig. 101 Turning over and folding up using Break Arm Style.

Chuang Tzu refers to '*Zhen Ren*', meaning 'True Person', someone who has transformed himself through Taoist practices such as TCC, and who is therefore capable of giving a true transmission of such practices. He says that their breathing came deep and silently; breathing from a True Man coming from his heels, while other men generally breathe from their throats. Here the emphasis is on correct breathing leading to a physical transformation and improvement.

Conditioning training and practice of form and Tai Chi Nei Kung are necessary for our actions to follow our intention, and for the breath to follow our actions, otherwise we will be sluggish and unco-ordinated. Such training also builds stamina so that we can comfortably continue to move.

*By constantly developing the Qi there is no evil.
By using the curve to gather the Jin
there is more than a sufficiency.*

These two sentences in Chinese are an interesting contrast. The term '*Zhi*', which

I have translated as 'constantly', can also mean 'straight'. It contrasts with the curve used to gather the *Jin*, just as the phrase 'there is no evil' contrasts with 'there is more than a sufficiency'. Everything is as it should be: deep breathing develops a sense of calm, and the force is more than enough to deal with the opponent. It is essential constantly to develop the *Qi* to give us the requisite level of stamina and breath control to practise TCC effectively. *Jin* is an elastic type of force, and is often deployed by using Yin in one half of a circle to defend and Yang in the other half to strike. When delivering *Jin* we don't lock the joints because this makes our movements stiff and causes long-term damage; this is also a physical manifestation of the dot of Yang in the Yin half, and the dot of Yin in the Yang half of the Tai Chi motif. This is what enables us to change.

The Xin (mind) acts as the commander;
The Qi acts as the flag;
The waist acts as the banner.

Chuang Tzu said the body, with its hundred parts, nine openings and six viscera, must have a true ruler. The ruler is the *Xin* (mind). When we do a technique we focus mind and body: this is the use of *Yi* (intent). The body, like an army, must immediately obey orders. Whether in defence or attack, immediately we wish to do something, then there is respiration and turn, like an order being issued and passed on through the chain of command in an army. However, I disagree with the Classic here; many martial arts teachers tell students to turn the waist or hips, when what is required is rotation of the spinal column.

First seek to expand (open), then seek to be compact (close).
Thus you reach fine work neatly done.

Beginners tend to exaggerate movements because they lack co-ordination and balance; with correction and practice their movements become more compact and refined. With an opponent our strategy should be to add force to his attacks and make them over-extended, while keeping our own movements compact. In many TCC styles the student progresses from a large frame form, to a medium frame form, and finally to a small frame or fine form. Taken to extremes, this can produce very poor work indeed. A notorious case was the late Gong-yi, son of the famous Wu Jian-quan, who produced a small frame form where the kicks were below knee height and in which the Snake failed to 'Creep Down' very far. I once had an animated discussion on this topic with American internal martial arts master Bruce Frantzis, and remain unconvinced by his assertion that the smaller the external movement, the more is happening internally. It is an easy claim to make, and a hard one to prove.

Older people and the sick find it harder to make large movements and to do the forms in an athletic manner, so their techniques tend to be understated; at the other extreme, modern Wushu TCC performers tend to over-extend and damage backs and knees.

It is also said:
First in the Xin (mind), then in the body.
The abdomen is spongy; the Qi is
hoarded to enter the bones;
The Shen (spirit) is at ease
and the body is tranquil.
This must be deeply engraved
on the Xin (mind).

The phrase 'it is also said…' is an example of formula (*jue*), a literary device to indicate that what follows is a later addition to the original text, perhaps by the same writer, but more likely by a later master.

Chuang Tzu said that if the spirit is used without rest, it becomes weary, then exhausted. If the mind is not relaxed, the body cannot relax. This is why we don't just go straight into the practice of the form and Tai Chi Nei Kung, but perform preparatory movements to develop mental focus. Many forms start with 'Tai Chi at Rest (*Wu Chi*)' followed by 'Tai Chi Ready Style (*Tai Chi*)' and only then 'Beginning Style'. This preparation acts as a series of triggers to focus the mind and prepare the body for the journey that is the form (*see* Figs 73 and 74).

'The abdomen is spongy' means that there is no tension there, and so it is easier for the diaphragm to move downwards to enable the lungs to take in more oxygen (*Qi*), making the circulation stronger and effecting a gentle massage of the internal organs. Tai Chi Nei Kung training enables the practitioner to take blows to the body including the abdomen, not because it is hard but because it absorbs the blows like a sponge.

The long bones in the body contain cavities. These cavities are filled with bone marrow, which produces blood cells. However, with age and decreasing activity the marrow decreases in vigour and consists mainly of fat. Joints are where two or more bones meet. They can be immovable (fibrous joints), as is the case with the bones of the skull; slightly movable, as is the case with the ribs, which are connected to the sternum by cartilage and with the vertebrae; or they can allow free movement (synovial joints). Synovial joints require synovial fluid to lubricate the joint cavity, pass on nutrients to the joint, and remove waste products. Production of this fluid depends on the physical activity of the joint and so inactivity causes a deficiency of synovial fluid, which in turn causes stiffening and creaking in the joint.

Qi being hoarded to enter the bones refers to regular practice of TCC, leading to improved respiration, causing in turn improved circulation as well as joint manipulation. It is common in TCC to experience a cracking sound as the joints are manipulated by exercise. This physical activity leads to increased production of synovial fluid and helps the bone marrow to maintain the production of blood cells. In turn this makes the body and mind feel at ease.

Many doctors are unhelpful to patients suffering from sprains and fractures induced by martial arts injuries, and often merely advise rest. One of my students, Dr Mike Webb, a medical researcher, provided me with a variety of research from American, Japanese and European sources, which shows that resistance training and high intensity strength exercises are an effective method of maintaining or even increasing bone mass density and muscle mass in different age groups.

Australian, American and Taiwanese studies further showed that TCC exercise produced cardio-respiratory benefits, improvements in posture control, and balance in those who practised it, as compared with sedentary control groups who did not.

Always remember, once there is movement,
there is nothing that does not move.
Once there is stillness there is
nothing that is not still.

All parts of the body should start and finish a movement together. This is the key to using total body force. Many students make the mistake of watching the arms of the instructors, but in TCC we do not defend and counter with the arms, but with the whole body; there is little independent arm movement. Stillness refers here to some Tai Chi Nei Kung exercises that, though static, combine body strengthening for martial purposes, self-defence, therapeutic and meditative aspects. When performing these exercises we should not arbitrarily move about, although the exercises themselves, particularly in the beginning and when performed for a long time, may cause the body to vibrate or shake. This is natural and we should not be concerned about it, but should keep the body relaxed, and the mind alert. This type of training gives us the mental stillness to analyse and deal with problems in a calm and unemotional way.

When moving back and forth,
The Qi sticks to the back,
It amasses and enters the spine.
Internally it strengthens the Jingshen (vigour);
Externally one exhibits peaceful ease.

Good respiration leads to good circulation, which 'strengthens the vigour' and leaves one exhibiting 'peaceful ease'. *Jing* (vital essence) and *Shen* (spiritual essence) together suggest 'vigour', or latent physical and mental energy. This improvement in circulation and respiration, combined with postural and alignment correction, helps to stimulate the central and autonomic nervous systems, and hence the brain.

This is also a direct reference to Taoist Internal Alchemy methods, where *Qi* is supposed to travel up the spine to nourish the brain – however, I have a number of reservations about the way these practices have been exploited by teachers of so-called sexual *Qi Gong*. Either they have been taught wrongly, or they have forgotten correct practice methods, or their practice is inherently dangerous or does not mix with their other esoteric practices. In Hong Kong I knew several Chinese people admitted to Castle Peak Psychiatric Hospital after having trained in such practices. Despite having received treatment, it was quite clear that they were not all right. Correct practice will help in the production of *Qi Jing Shen*, the Three Treasures of Internal Alchemy leading to greater well-being; incorrect practice can do physical and mental harm.

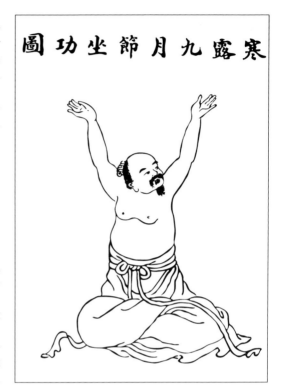

Fig. 102 Sitting *Qigong*.

Move the way a cat walks.
Mobilize the Jin as if reeling silk from a cocoon.

Cats seem to be relaxed, but are extremely alert, ready for any sudden danger, and are able to move nimbly in any direction in reaction to any eventuality. If silk is jerked when reeled from a cocoon, it is liable to break; if it is pulled too softly, nothing happens. By analogy *Jin* should be neither over- nor under-extended. If under-extended, the *Jin* will lack penetration; if over-extended, it will be difficult to change to do something else. Largely through the Chen clan, a plethora of pseudo science has grown up around 'reeling silk' and many books refer to 'reeling silk *Jin*' as if this were a separate type of *Jin*. The late TCC historian, Wu Tu-nan, among others, ridiculed this practice. Chen 'Reeling Silk' is simply coiling and uncoiling the limbs and torso, a practice common to many martial arts. This smooth, circular and continuous use of *Jin* is shown in Figs 99 and 100.

The body and the Yi (intent) are entirely
concentrated on the Jingshen (vigour),
Not on the Qi.
If on the Qi,
Then there is stagnation.
If there is Qi then there is no strength (Li).
If there is no Qi then there is great strength.
The Qi is like the wheel of a chariot;
The waist is like an axle.

Concentrating on the *Jingshen* requires us to prepare for practice by composing the mind and ignoring external distractions. Hence, we have triggers in the forms and in the ritual manner of Tai Chi Nei Kung practice enabling us to do this; such training in concentration, combined with regular practice of self-defence applications, enables us to 'switch on' when attacked.

Practice should be vigorous, which implies that stances should be sufficiently deep, movements should be lively – even slow ones – and there should be meaning and therefore intent behind each technique. This makes it necessary to familiarize ourselves with the purpose of each technique.

If we concentrate on the *Qi*, we are concentrating on what our body is doing, rather than dealing with what the opponent is trying to do to us. Many say, 'Breathe naturally' – but how? We shouldn't have to think about when to breathe in or out; the movements will control all this. Where there is

insufficient stamina we will inevitably be very concerned with the *Qi*; we will puff and pant, and there will indeed be no strength because the movements will become disordered and unco-ordinated, as well as lacking in focus. However, when someone's breath is inaudible despite great exertion, then there is indeed great strength and stamina. This is what is meant by 'if ... no *Qi* then there is great strength'.

Strength is one of the components necessary to strike or throw an opponent or to thrust with a spear, but the trick is not to use just brute force. We use educated force in TCC, a combination of strength, speed, weight, timing, intent and technique. This gives the lie to those who say that only practising the form, some pushing hands and self-defence applications is sufficient for fighting, and underlines the importance of conditioning training.

Some instructors aver that we should breathe in or out at certain points. There is a tendency to breathe out on expansive movements and to breathe in on contracting ones, but no more than that. Some movements are short, some long, some fast and some slow. The requirements of the movements dictate the breathing.

Movement and breath are one, and depend on one another like a wheel depends on an axle in order to propel a chariot. Movement is directed not by the waist, but by centre line rotation, and correct movement promotes correct breathing. Once we are relaxed and breathing in and out through the nose, with the tip of the tongue pressed against the roof of the mouth, breathing is not something we need to think about.

10 Classic 4: Song of the Thirteen Tactics (*Shi San Shi Ge*)

This is the least substantial of the five major essays that make up the TCC Classics. Although this classic is entitled *Song of the Thirteen Tactics* (said to be another name for TCC), it fails to mention any of the said tactics by name. The text contains references to Internal Alchemy, an emphasis on the use of the waist, and the repeated mention of the *Yi* (intent) and even (three times) of *Kung Fu* in the sense of effort or energy. Internal Alchemy was not universally approved of even by Taoist writers. Chuang Tzu ridiculed adepts who wished for the longevity of Peng Tzu (a Chinese Methuselah), blowing and breathing open-mouthed; inhaling and exhaling; expelling the old breath, and taking in new.

Perhaps the most useful passage is the one emphasizing the necessity for private tuition to learn the art properly. This type of personal tuition is a fundamental consequence of the traditional master–disciple relationship, and is another example of the gulf in understanding between most present-day practitioners of TCC and those few who had, or have, such a master–disciple relationship.

The message of the Classic is that practising the Thirteen Tactics will aid our development in a therapeutic, alchemical and martial way. We should not allow ourselves to be distracted while employing our mind, and we don't just use the arms and legs arbitrarily.

Though physical practice is emphasized, the writer makes clear that this is not enough by itself and that study and thought are indispensable if we are to achieve a high level. As with Classic 3, this suggests influences such as the *Nei Ye* (Inward Training) and Complete Reality School texts.

TCC Classic 4

The thirteen general tactics must
not be underestimated.
Make the source of fulfilling the
Yi (intent) at the waist.
During the changes and turnings of void
and substantial, you must maintain the Yi.
The Qi circulates throughout the body
without the slightest obstacle.
There is stillness even if there is movement;
When there is movement there is stillness.
In accordance with the opponent
my changes appear mysterious.
Every tactic lives in the Xin (mind),
the principle is to use the Yi (intent).
In the attainment of perfection do
not waste Kung Fu (effort).
Carve and carve again into the Xin
(mind) it should be on the waist.
Internally the abdomen is relaxed
and still and the Qi ascends,
When the Wei Lu (coccyx) is Zhong
Zheng (centrally correct), the Shen
(spirit) connects with the headtop.

The whole body feels light and agile
when the headtop is suspended.
Be meticulous and keep the Xin
(mind) on enquiring into the art.
Freely contract and extend,
open and close and listen.
To go through the gate and be led along
the path oral instruction is necessary.
Kung Fu (effort) is unceasing.
Cultivate the method yourself.
Let us enquire into what acts as the
rule for the body (in all this):
The Yi (intent) and the Qi are the rulers;
The bones and the flesh are the officials.
Think and enquire where does
the final purpose lie?
It lies in seeking longevity and
keeping a youthful appearance.
This is a song of 140 characters.
Every character has a clear meaning
and there is nothing omitted.
If you don't enquire into the subject in this way,
You vainly waste Kung Fu (time
and energy) and heave a sigh.

Commentary

The thirteen general tactics must
not be underestimated.
Make the source of fulfilling the
Yi (intent) at the waist.
During the changes and turnings of void
and substantial, you must maintain the Yi.
The Qi circulates throughout the body
without the slightest obstacle.
There is stillness even if there is movement;
In movement yet there is stillness.

The Thirteen Tactics are dealt with in more detail in Classic 2, but in short they consist of eight methods of using force, which are identified with the *Ba Gua* (Eight Trigrams) and five directions for stepping, which are identified with the Five Elements.

When wishing to make any movement, the way to achieve it is by turning not the waist, but the centre line. Constantly we extend and contract the limbs and shift the weight in different directions while the abdomen contracts and expands (that is, *Qi* is sent to and from the *Dan Tian*). Doing this slowly and smoothly helps *Qi* to circulate throughout the body. TCC methods of training the centre line are found in pushing hands and Tai Chi Nei Kung, as well as in the hand and weapon forms. Waist is a misnomer: it is the use of centre line theory and the spinal column that is meant here.

The *Yi* (intent) must be maintained at all times, whether your techniques or your opponent's are void (feints) or substantial (genuine attacks). TCC has many techniques, such as 'Flick the Whip' and 'Running Thunder Hand' used as feints, or to bridge the gap between ourselves and an opponent, as with the jab of Western boxing. What we practise most is what we are most likely to use; these are techniques I emphasize for self-defence. In free pushing hands and grappling, the intent is to maintain our own balance and concentration while disturbing that of the opponent. In TCC forms, and Tai Chi Nei Kung training, there is little or no independent head movement; this helps us to develop peripheral vision so we are aware of, but not influenced by external distractions. Regarding stillness and movement, even if we do not seem to be moving externally, the mind remains alert and the breath smooth, though inaudible. The face is in repose when practising form; this is not necessarily so in the practice of weapons and self-defence. These ideas are also borrowed from Lao Tzu: 'I go to the limit to reach emptiness, I hold firmly to stillness...' (*Tao Te Ching* Ch. 16).

In accordance with the opponent
my changes appear mysterious.

*Every tactic lives in the Xin (mind),
the principle is to use the Yi (intent).
In the attainment of perfection do
not waste Kung Fu (effort).
Carve and carve again into the Xin
(mind) it should be on the waist.*

Because TCC is a counterattacking method we often pre-empt attacks or give back to the opponent his own force, using the centre line (not waist) in defence and counter attack, no matter which combination of the Thirteen Tactics we deploy. So the opponent finds his attacks unexpectedly diverted and countered. The tactics must become second nature and must be done with intent, if they are to be effective. Wasting effort means that when you train, you must do the right type of training. Form training in isolation is useless for self-defence; pushing hands and applications practice with a variety of partners is essential.

Concentrating the mind on the waist means that though the arms are intercepting, redirecting and striking, this is almost invariably done by turning the body so that we are using total body force. The use of the phrase, 'Carve and carve again…' is not accidental and refers to the 'Uncarved Block', which is a metaphor for *Wu Chi* (No Ultimate). These two concepts of infinite potentiality both appear in Chapter 28 of Lao Tzu's *Tao Te Ching*.

A sculptor or carpenter cannot immediately carve fine detail on a block of wood or stone, but first works on the broad outline; so it is with martial arts. Many teachers confuse students by over-teaching or teaching what is beyond them, rather than taking a step-by-step approach. It is important to stress repeatedly key points in technique, and for the student to build a muscle memory by repeated practice of them. With the third level in Tai Chi Nei Kung some techniques are repeated more than a thousand times, and when doing conditioning training I regularly used to practise Running Thunder Hand with light weights, doing more than 3,000 repetitions in twenty minutes.

*Internally the abdomen is relaxed
and still and the Qi ascends,
When the Wei Lu (coccyx) is Zhong
Zheng (centrally straight), the Shen
(spirit) connects with the headtop.
The whole body feels light and agile
when the headtop is suspended.*

This is another attempt to link TCC practice with the Internal Alchemy rejuvenation practice of sending the *Qi* or the *Jing* up the spine to nourish the brain, where it is converted into *Shen*. TCC emphasizes correct alignment of the spine, which should be straight, but not necessarily erect at all times. The coccyx is tucked in, so that there is a straight line from the crown of the head down the spine to the coccyx; this alignment helps the function of the central nervous system, which runs through the spinal column; Figs 103 and 104 respectively show this alignment in back stance and forward stance.

A disproportionate number of TCC books have been written by practitioners of Cheng Man-ching style, because he was the first Chinese TCC teacher to become famous in the West. Certain parts of the Classics, such as this one, have not been correctly explained, many of these writers insisting that the body should be upright and erect at all times during TCC practice. However, not only are famous masters from other styles often neither upright nor erect, but even Cheng himself, in books and films, can be seen to be inclined when performing certain techniques.

Taken separately, *Zhong* means centre or central, and *Zheng* means 'straight'/'correct' and (sometimes) 'upright'. In the

95

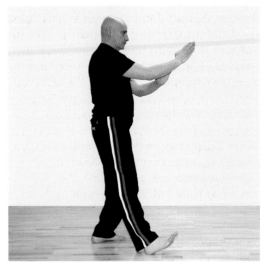

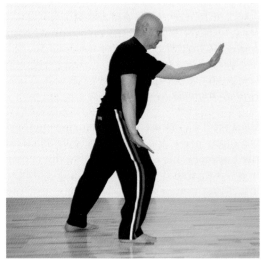

Fig. 103 Seven Stars.

Fig. 104 Brush Knee Twist Step.

commentary of Classic 3 we had a wide-ranging discussion of *Zhong Zheng* ('centrally straight'/'correct'). With regard to body alignment, this term is often narrowly interpreted as 'exactly upright', but nobody is actually doing this, and it is clear that the broader interpretation of 'centrally straight' is more accurate.

The head is heavy, so if it is not properly aligned, we will feel uncomfortable and it will be difficult to move easily – the body will not feel light and agile. 'Suspended headtop' does *not* require that the head is positioned at all times as if vertically suspended from the ceiling. The reason for the emphasis on a straight back is to improve balance and posture, and to allow the lungs to expand as much as possible. In addition, the discs of cartilage between the vertebrae act as shock absorbers, preventing the transmission of jolts caused by movement to the base of the skull, and they can only do this effectively if there is correct alignment in the first place. Some styles, such as my own, put more than 90 per cent of the weight on to the front foot when in a front stance. Doing this requires

the torso to be inclined further forwards than in other styles, thus stretching and re-aligning the spinal column, releasing pressure on the discs, and stimulating the central nervous system. There are some TCC fascists who strive to be physically upright at all times, and as a result the spine is always compressed.

Be meticulous and keep the Xin
(mind) on enquiring into the art.
Freely contract and extend,
open and close and listen.
To go through the gate and be led along
the path oral instruction is necessary.
Kung Fu (effort) is unceasing.
Cultivate the method yourself.

The first sentence tells us to train in an aware and analytical way. Many martial arts practitioners go through their forms without thinking about what they are doing, the inevitable result of not knowing the applications of the movements.

The second sentence paraphrases Lao Tzu's 'To shrink something, you must first stretch it. To weaken something, you must first strengthen it. To take from something, you must first give to it…The soft and weak will overcome the hard and strong' (*Tao Te Ching* Ch. 36). Usually we contract to defend, and extend when striking. We open when performing rising, expansive movements – for example, the rib cage opens, thereby stretching the lungs and internal organs – and we close when performing sinking, contracting movements. This makes movements better co-ordinated and therefore stronger, as well as producing a pumping action, which enhances the respiration and circulation. The hand form is done relatively slowly so that these actions can combine with the effect of gravity.

'To go through the gate and be led along the path' refers to a student becoming a disciple or inside-the-door student after undergoing the *Bai Shi* (respect teacher/teachings) ritual initiation ceremony with his master in front of a portrait of Chang San-feng, the founder of TCC. After this, being now a disciple, he is given advanced training methods, including Tai Chi Nei Kung. Such instruction is private and not given in open classes. Few teachers now have the knowledge required for this type of instruction, and many Western practitioners feel that such élitism has no place in their liberal world of sharing ideas and information. Yet we have the strange situation where only a handful of people have been trained in Cheng Man-ching's Nei Kung system (though it is not a Tai Chi Nei Kung), while this is one of the more prevalent TCC styles in Europe and North America, and no one from this style seems to complain about their exclusion.

Oral instruction includes the mnemonic TCC Classics and, in my own school at least, the recitation of a mantra. It also includes tuition in specific skills or concepts such as Six Secret Words. I retain *Bai Shi* in my school, not for reasons of secrecy, but because I believe that people should show a degree of dedication and sincerity before moving on to more advanced concepts and more vital

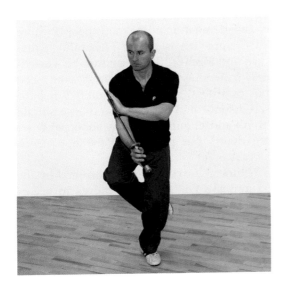

Fig. 105 Contracting/closing: Sparrow Hawk turns round.

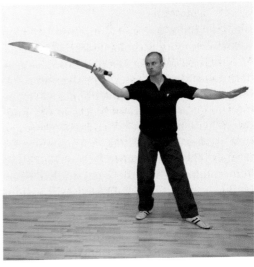

Fig. 106 Extending/opening: *Peng* spreads Wings.

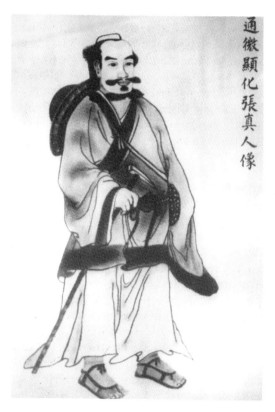

通微顯化張真人像

Fig. 107 Chang San-feng.

credibility: it is not a matter of spending money, but of not wasting time and energy. I know many practitioners who, after more than twenty years' practice, have little to show for it except a few forms and 'the big push'. Don't be like them.

Let us enquire into what acts
as the rule for the body:
The Yi (intent) and the Qi (vital
force) are the rulers;
The bones and the flesh are the officials.
Think and enquire, where does
the final purpose lie?
It lies in seeking longevity and
keeping a youthful appearance.
This is a song of 140 characters.
Every character has a clear meaning
and there is nothing omitted.
If you don't enquire into the subject in this way,
You vainly waste Kung Fu (time
and energy) and heave a sigh.

'Let us enquire...' suggests that this is another formula (*Jue*), perhaps added as a postscript by some later master. This passage is a condemnation of the many people whose TCC approach is to use physicality rather than intelligence. They cannot be considered 'rulers' as the physicality is controlled not by intent, but by emotion. As regards self-defence and pushing hands, we should 'think and enquire' not just about what we are doing, but also about the opponent's actions.

Ultimately everything is controlled by the *Yi* and the *Qi*. The body moves in accordance with the *Yi*, the *Qi* flows and the rest follows. The emphasis in this Classic is on correct principles of practice and *Qi* circulation, although there is also a short reference to dealing with an opponent. This final paragraph mentions an ancient obsession with the Chinese: longevity. Chuang Tzu said, 'You must be still and pure, not subjecting

training. PhDs are not conferred on high school dropouts. Regular incorrect practice of *Nei/Qi Gong/Kung* systems is notoriously harmful, and even correct practice can cause initial problems if the practitioner is suffering from certain types of illness or old injuries. What Chinese refer to as 'true transmission' is vital: personal tuition from an expert teacher. The last sentence follows Lao Tzu's admonition: 'When the best student hears about the way (Tao), he practises it assiduously' (*Tao Te Ching* Ch. 41).

There is now a plethora of oral instruction available on the internet either from pimple-faced, teenage scribblers who can't find a girlfriend, or burnt-out old soaks entering the second half of a wasted life. If you want instruction, find someone who has the body to toil, not agitating the vital force – then you may live long.'

Taoists refer to the concept of 'Long life, not old', and the aim was to live a long life without the infirmities that normally afflict the aged. They attempted to achieve this through the physiological alchemy methods that they developed. TCC, as well as being a martial art, contains many of the principles, and the TCC Classics contain much of the jargon of Taoist Internal Alchemy theory.

The 'final purpose' can only be achieved by serious study and practice of Internal Alchemy. In TCC this is by slow practice of the hand form and Tai Chi Nei Kung. '*Kung Fu*' here means time and energy, and the emphasis is on doing the right kind of training. The *Yi* and the *Qi* stimulate and strengthen the bones and flesh. Many studies have shown the benefits of exercise in general and TCC in particular on people of different age groups, especially the elderly; benefits include improvements in balance and posture, as well as maintenance or enhancement of bone mass density.

It is a matter of lifestyle, too. Yang Zhenduo, fourth generation master of Yang family Tai Chi Chuan and son of Yang Cheng-fu, was interviewed by Pierre-Yves Bénoliel, the editor, in issue 5, October 2004, of the French martial arts magazine *Dragon*. Pierre-Yves asked Yang under what circumstances his father, Yang Cheng-fu, died at the age of fifty-three. There is no good answer to this killer question. Yang replied that his father was in Guangdong, South China. He was a big, strong man weighing 138kg (more than 300lb). Because of the heat, he perspired profusely, causing a kind of eczema of his genitalia. In Hong Kong there is a well known malady called 'Hong Kong Foot', a fungus between the toes due to sweat, and his nephew proposed that he use the foot ointment, so he rubbed the product on his genitalia. The result was catastrophic because the product was toxic, and caused a huge swelling of his genitalia. He was urgently taken to Shanghai (a considerable distance), but medicine was not as developed as it is today, and no one was able to save him.

11 Classic 5: The Fighter's Song (*Da Shou Ge*)

The *Da* (hit) *Shou* (hands) *Ge* (song) is often rendered in English as the 'Song of Pushing Hands'. This translation is both incorrect and misleading. *Tui Shou* (pushing hands) is not mentioned in either the title or the text, although some of the concepts mentioned can be applied, or are trained, in pushing hands. The term 'pushing hands' does not appear in any of the TCC Classics, and is inaccurate because many of the exercises it describes do not necessarily involve either pushing or the use of the hands.

Da Shou Ge can be translated literally as the 'Song of Striking Hands', but in Chinese a '*Da Shou*' is also a fighter, so I have rendered this Classic as the 'Fighter's Song', which is an apt description of the material. We don't know who wrote this text, but he/they certainly knew about fighting, though there are many references to 'internal' elements such as soft, light and agile and keeping the intent unbroken. If there really is a big difference between internal and external martial arts, this text sets it out.

TCC Classic 5

Peng, Lu, Ji and An must be taken seriously.
Up and down accompany one another and
the opponent finds it difficult to enter.
Let him attack with great force,
Use four taels to displace a thousand catties

Entice the opponent into the void
(emptiness) harmonize and promptly discharge
Adhere, be continuous, be soft, follow,
don't break contact or resist.
Cai, Lie, Zhou and Kao are
even more amazing,
When using them there is no
need to think about it.
If you can be light and agile you
then can understand Jin (force)
Achieve it inside a circle, not with
hands and feet disorganized.
Furthermore, the secret/trick is:
If the opponent doesn't move,
I don't move.
If the opponent moves a little,
Then I move first.
Seeming relaxed, but don't relax;
Be prepared to move, but don't move.
The Jin is broken, but the
Yi (intent) is unbroken.

Commentary

Peng, Lu, Ji and An must be taken seriously.
Up and down accompany one another and
the opponent finds it difficult to enter.

The Eight Forces are dealt with in Classic 1. This commentary illustrates them using typical TCC fighting techniques in a way that may be unfamiliar to some TCC practitioners. These forces can be defensive or offensive, and soft or hard.

In using *Peng*, we can raise the arms to divert the opponent's hands up or to upper-cut him. Fig. 108 shows both defensive and offensive *Peng* applied simultaneously in an application of 'Turn around Swing Fist'.

With *Lu*, the hands come from above or from the outside or inside to divert the opponent's attack to the left or right. *Lu* is often followed by *An*, where we suddenly press or push downwards. Figs 109–111 show the use of *Lu*, *Cai*, *An* in an application of 'Step Back to Beat the Tiger'.

Peng is often followed by *Ji*, where force is used in a straight line, such as a direct push or palm strike to the opponent's chest. Fig. 112 shows the use of *Peng Ji* in an application of 'Under Elbow See Fist'.

The 'on guard' position in Chinese martial arts is sometimes referred to as the door or gate. Using immediate defence and counter-attack at different levels – such as defending the head and countering below said defence – makes it difficult for the opponent to 'enter'

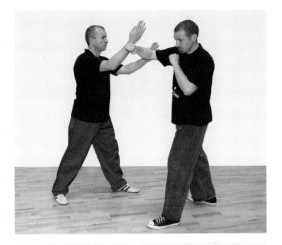

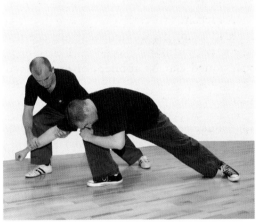

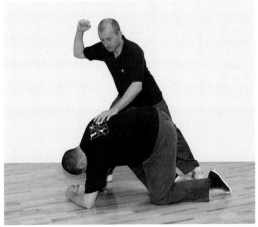

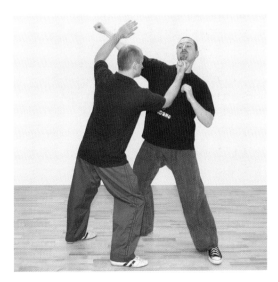

Fig. 108 *Peng* using Turn Around Swing Fist.

Figs 109–111 *Lu*, *Cai*, *An* using Step Back to Beat the Tiger.

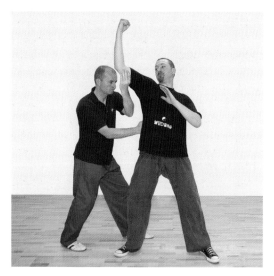

Fig. 112 *Peng Ji* using Under Elbow See Fist.

that door – that is, he cannot penetrate our defences.

Let him attack with great force,
Use four taels to displace a thousand catties
Entice the opponent into the void (emptiness)
harmonize and promptly discharge

Lao Tzu and Chuang Tzu both talk about *Wu Wei* and Lao Tzu even says, '*Wu wei er bu wei*' (non-action till nothing not acted) (*Tao Te Ching* Ch. 48), and '*Wei wu wei*' ('act without acting') (*Tao Te Ching* Ch. 63).

Wu Wei is often wrongly interpreted as 'doing nothing'. Beat movement author, martial artist and philosopher, Alan Watts, gives an excellent explanation: for him, *Wu Wei* is like being in a boat on a river and wanting to go upstream. An arduous solution is to attempt to row against the current; the *Wu Wei* solution is to put up a sail and use the wind. It is not about doing nothing, but to harmonize and avoid conflict with the elements that are present. The metaphor of using only four taels to displace a massive force is exactly *Wu Wei* in action.

TCC uses Yin to overcome Yang. Instead of using a hard block against the opponent's attack, we intercept and redirect it simultaneously using footwork and/or body evasion so that we are not encountering the force head on. In so doing his force is confronted by nothing but emptiness – 'the void' – and thus he is unbalanced and unable to defend himself. After harmonizing with the attack we immediately discharge or counterattack – thought and action are trained to be as one. This is what makes TCC an ideal method of self-defence for lighter or smaller individuals faced with larger opponents who employ brute force.

Adhere, be continuous, be soft, follow,
don't break contact or resist.

These are five strategies for close-quarter fighting, which we can practise in pushing hands training. Some of the strategies overlap to a degree.

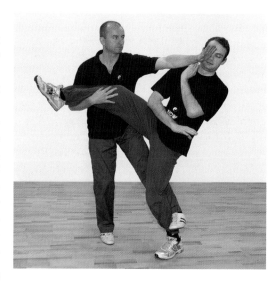

Fig. 113 Sweep Lotus Leg – using *Peng, Cai, An, Lie.*

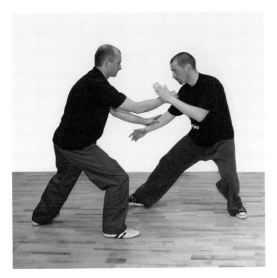

Fig. 114 Free pushing hands.

Nian means 'to stick' or 'adhere'. Once the distance between us and the opponent has been bridged and we are at close quarters, *Nian* requires that our hands or arms should at all times be in contact with the opponent's hands and arms. When at close quarters with an opponent we have very little time in which to react. By the time the eyes have sent a message to the brain, and the brain has issued orders to the body, it is often too late. We therefore rely on 'listening' ability, TCC jargon for sensitivity through physical contact with an opponent. Having such contact enables us to control the opponent, making it difficult for him to strike us, and enabling us to use his arms as levers to unbalance him.

Lian means 'continuity' and 'connection', so defence and response are not separate movements, and if one defence or counter is unsuccessful or insufficient, it is immediately followed by another. In a number of instances in the form, one technique follows another for reasons of self-defence; if the first move is unsuccessful, or if there was more than one opponent, then the second technique is used.

Mian means 'cotton' and is therefore synonymous with soft. Softness is necessary for successful listening, but only a fool would hit softly. It takes more energy to be stiff and hard, it is also easier and quicker to change from soft to hard than from hard to soft, though the latter is an important skill that many TCC practitioners do not have. Ideally we should be soft unless, and until, we have to be hard.

Sui is often translated as 'yielding', which has the connotation of going backwards, but this is inaccurate and the term should more accurately be translated as 'following'. Following requires moving in a complementary way to the opponent: thus if he steps forwards, we step back or round; if he goes back, we step forwards or in. Likewise while adhering our arms follow his direction of force.

Bu Diu Ding means 'not to break contact' or 'to resist'. If we break contact, not only can we not 'listen', but we are in imminent danger of being hit by the arm/s that we have released. If we resist by using force directly against force, not only are we wasting energy, but we also can't listen effectively. This emphasizes the three-step process of *Ting Jin* (listen for *Jin* – that is for the opponent to attack), *Hua Jin* (redirect the opponent's *Jin* with our defensive *Jin*) and *Fa Jin* (discharge *Jin*), which we discussed in the commentary to Classic 2.

*Cai, Lie, Zhou and Kao are
even more amazing,
When using them there is no
need to think about it.*

Cai is 'to pluck' and involves uprooting the opponent; often it is preceded by *Peng* or *Lu*.

Lie is the use of spiralling force, where the opponent's technique or our counter is spiralled into, or away from him.

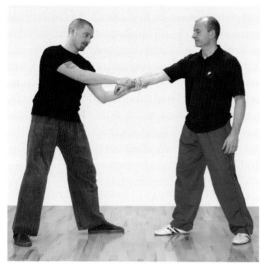

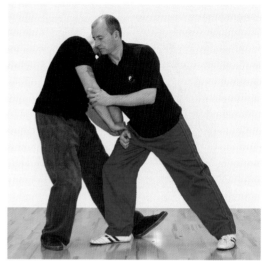

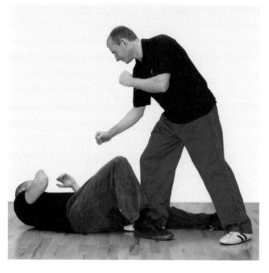

CLOCKWISE FROM TOP LEFT: Figs 115–117 *Sui* – following the opponent's force and adding to it.

Zhou is the use of the forearm or elbow.

Kao, meaning 'to lean', is the use of the shoulder or body to barge the opponent.

These four forces must be trained so that they are spontaneous and natural responses. As with the first four forces, they can be defensive or offensive, and soft or hard. They are slightly more difficult to apply, and in the case of *Cai* and *Lie* are somewhat more subtle than the other forces.

As with bare-hand techniques, TCC weapons such as spear, sabre and sword are each credited with Eight Forces or methods of use. Again this is somewhat artificial; mainly the terms used are different to those of the bare-hand techniques.

If you can be light and agile you
then can understand Jin,
Achieve it inside a circle, not with
hands and feet disorganized.

Understanding *Jin* is being able to *Ting*, *Hua*, *Fa Jin* (Listen for, Transform and Discharge Force: *see* Figs 79–81, pages 71–2). *Jin* can be soft or hard, long or short, is elastic and dynamic, and can be defined as educated or trained force as opposed to crude brute force. The circular nature of many TCC techniques makes it easy to effect the transformation from soft to hard, from Yin to Yang. This also requires the use of total body force, hands and feet moving in unison.

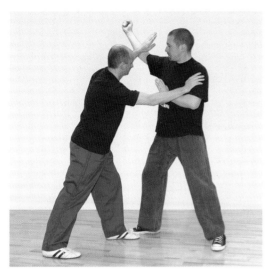 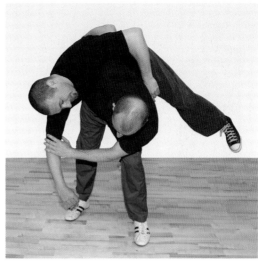

Figs 118 and 119 *Lu* and *Ji* in Grasping Bird's Tail, and *Cai* in White Crane Flaps Wings.

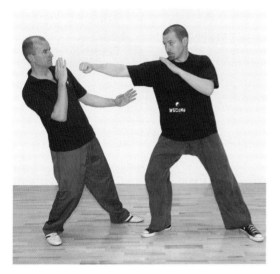 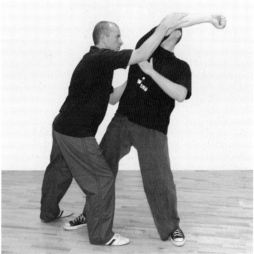

Figs 120 and 121 *Lie* in Fair Lady Works at Shuttle.

Furthermore, the formula/trick is:
If the opponent doesn't move,
I don't move.
If the opponent moves a little
Then I move first.

I have translated '*Jue*' as formula/trick; it can also mean method. As with the 'it is also said…' at the end of Classic 3, this is a post-script that may have been written by some later master and tacked on at the end of the

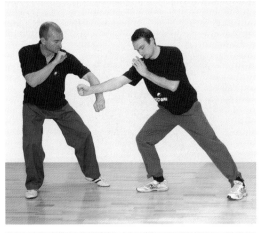
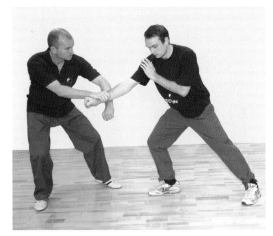
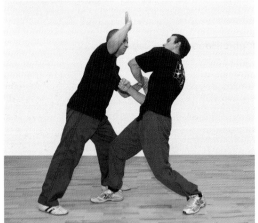
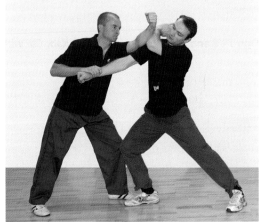
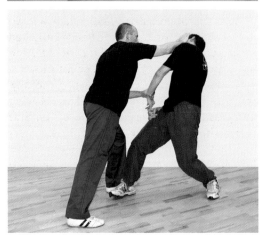

CLOCKWISE FROM TOP LEFT: Figs 122–126 *Zhou, Cai, An, Lie, Ji* with Swing the Fist.

text. It contains some of the most important self-defence concepts that have ever been written, and it needs detailed examination. The same ideas are also found in Taoism, 'Deal with a thing while it is still nothing' (*Tao Te Ching* Ch. 64).

The idea of stillness and motion in a martial sense appears in Huang Zong-xi's tombstone inscription for his master, Wang Zheng-nan: '…In the so-called Internal Family/School, (*Nei Jia*) stillness is used to control movement; when the opponent attacks then he is countered.' The idea is to react early to pre-empt an intended attack and neutralize it before it is fully launched. In sword duelling,

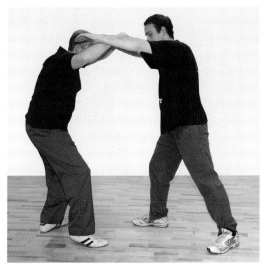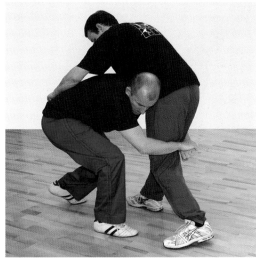

Figs 127 and 128 The use of *Peng, Kao, Cai* with Double Hands Seize Legs.

Chuang Tzu talks about moving after the opponent has started his attack, but beating him to the cut.

The concept of 'Stillness defeats motion' involves the seeming passivity of a clear mind (Yin) ready to match the motion (Yang) of an opponent. TCC is not usually an attacking method; it is a counterattacking method. If someone is committed to an attack, it is difficult for him to change his movement or his mind, and he is vulnerable to a counterattack. In TCC, we sometimes defend by attacking, either beating the opponent to the punch or using a feint to provoke him to move so that we can follow up with a counter once he is committed to his attack.

Self-defence is often poorly taught, and much poor stuff has been published on the subject. Often the defender in these productions only starts defending at a very late stage, when the opponent has already grabbed his arm or clothing or has fully launched his punch or kick. There are three timings: 'after the technique is on' is where we see that the opponent is going to attack us, he then does so, and we try to react after having been hit. This is too late. 'When the technique is on' is where we see the attack being launched, and we manage to avoid or redirect it, and hopefully counterattack. This is not ideal. 'Before the technique is on' is where we see that the opponent intends to attack us, and immediately counter with a pre-emptive strike or restraining technique. This is the ideal.

It is more effective, and certainly faster, to beat the opponent to the punch and to counter him before he has actually launched his attack. This requires great concentration and expert timing. 'If the opponent moves a little, then I move first.' Timing is the key, and too fast is as bad as too slow. Moving step pushing hands drills such as Seven Star Step, Nine Palace Step and Four Corners help to match our timing to a partner exactly. This is one of the first things I teach. In some karate styles evasion is not taught until the third Dan black belt level, a process that takes around eight years!

Seem relaxed, but don't relax
Be prepared to move, but don't move.

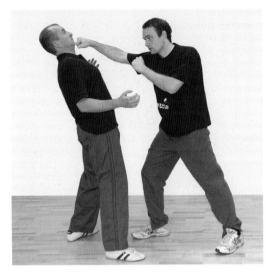

Fig. 129 Reacting after the technique is on.

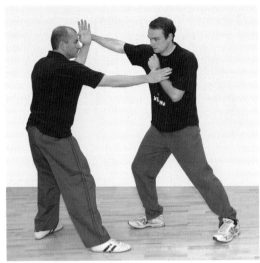

Fig. 130 Reacting when the technique is on.

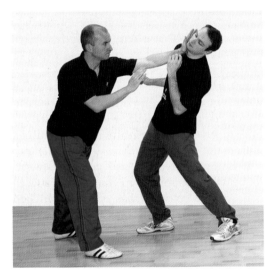

Fig. 131 Reacting before the technique is on.

The emphasis here is on alertness, concentration and natural posture, so that we are ready to move rapidly and smoothly in any direction, but only when it is necessary to move. It is important to be relaxed, but not limp. The same emphasis applies when we are practising pushing hands, applications or forms. 'Excellent as a soldier and not seeming martial. Excellent in fighting but not angry' (*Tao Te Ching* Ch. 68). In other words, we are ready to act in accord with the opponent.

The Jin is broken, but the
Yi (intent) is unbroken.

This key phrase has a double-edged meaning. When our *Jin*, whether defensive or offensive and whether successful or unsuccessful, is completed, we still retain the intent to defend or to counterattack as appropriate: our 'intent is unbroken'. Likewise, even if the opponent is under control, at any moment he may struggle or attack again; although for a particular instant his *Jin* is broken, he may still have the intent to attack us again. He can block our counter as in 'Swing the Fist' (Figs 122–126), so we change from hard to soft to control the blocking arm and follow up with another counter. We can also exploit his psychological state by pretending to resist his force and then suddenly giving way, or by applying force in one direction to draw the opponent into resisting, then suddenly changing the direction of our force.

We can train the spontaneity of this skill when we are practising free-style pushing hands or free fighting, because we don't know when the opponent will try to do something to us, and must ourselves be ready to follow one technique with another. I once had a street fight in Hong Kong where I hit my opponent with two full power groin kicks. When he tried to rush me a third time, I swept him and gave him a couple of punches to the temple to end the confrontation.

Another example of the need to maintain the intent is 'Recovery', a key concept in medieval European weapon training. After missing with one technique, whether accidentally or by design, one recovers into a guard, a parry or a follow-up. This same concept exists amongst skilled practitioners in every martial art. It is hardly mentioned in books on TCC, not because it is secret, but because most practitioners have never heard of it, far less know how to do it. Yet TCC forms are full of sequences designed to train such situations with a partner or partners. Among the explanations of *Classic of Boxing* postures in Part III, there are many examples of this concept.

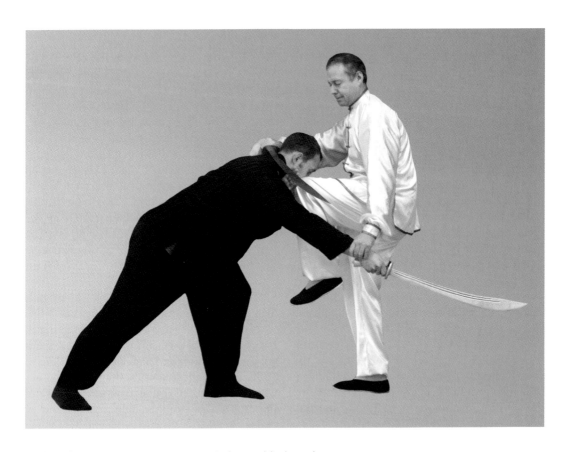

Author demonstrates a recovery technique with the sabre.

PART III
THE DUALITY OF *WEN WU*

I now turn to two key texts that represent the two extremes of the duality that is *wen wu*: the cultural/civil and the martial/military. Looking through the prism of these texts, we can understand the theory and practice of TCC more deeply, as well as shedding more light on the TCC Classics.

It is polarity rather than duality that we are more likely to encounter when dealing with the cultural and the martial. This is immediately obvious when we read the books of academic writers on TCC. They obviously have limited knowledge of the martial, but feel compelled to write about it; like eunuchs writing on the pleasures of love-making. Even Confucius, an extreme example some might think, of the cultural, advised young men to practice archery and charioteering, while the great poet, Li Bai, was a knight-errant who once wrote 'At fifteen, I loved the sword.' My own teacher, though without formal qualifications, wrote a number of ground-breaking books on TCC. The best people could and did and do practice both the cultural and the martial.

The first text we will examine is cultural, the *Tai Chi Diagram Explanation* by the Neo-Confucian philosopher, Zhou Dun-yi. The text contains symbolism, cosmogony and philosophy and is not directly martial,

although parallels exist with martial arts, meditative and Internal Alchemy practices.

The second text is martial, the *Classic of Boxing* by General Qi Ji-guang. Again there are parallels with TCC practice, but only with martial aspects and only to some degree.

These two very different men, living some five centuries apart, can be justly considered to personify respectively the cultural and the martial. The one was a leading scholar in what was a new age in Chinese philosophical thought. The other, General Qi Ji-guang, was a true hero and patriot who protected the Fujian coast from the depredations of Japanese pirates. In 2004, I visited his memorial temple in Fujian where his memory is still revered, although the flimsy sword on display is as likely to be that of General Qi as the battle-axe displayed in my own land is to be that that was used by Robert the Bruce to slay Sir Henry de Bohun at the battle of Bannockburn.

The texts are themselves 'classics' in their own right, and although they are not TCC texts as such, they are certainly source material. Necessarily my commentaries on them are mainly concerned with how they relate to TCC and so these commentaries are somewhat less detailed, but I trust no less useful than those that precede them.

12 Wen – Cultural: Zhou Dun-yi's *Tai Chi Diagram Explanation*

Zhou Dun-yi (1017–73) was a member of the Tai Chi Diagram Sect, which is often termed Neo-Confucian as they tried to connect the relationship of Man with Heaven above and Earth below through a re-examination of classical texts. He was an adept of Taoist physiological alchemy and so was someone who walked the walk and didn't just talk the talk; it is not known for sure whether or not he practised martial arts, but it would not be a surprise if he did.

There are many similarities between the concepts and terminology expressed in the '*Tai Chi Tu Shuo*' (*Tai Chi Diagram Explanation*) text and those at the beginning of Classic 2. It is useful to read the texts in parallel. '*Zhong Zheng*' (Centrally Correct), which is used in a martial and meditative sense in Classics 3 and 4, is used here in a metaphysical sense, hence the slightly different translation. The Five Elements appear in Zhou's text, but in a different order to the one given in Classic 1.

This text mixes ideas of cosmogony, duality, harmony and sophism from Mohism, Taoism, the Logicians and the Confucian School. It can be understood on a physical or metaphysical level. Zhou's Diagram was based on earlier work such as that of the great Taoist internal alchemist and philosopher, Chen Duan (906–89), who reputedly carved his *Wu Chi* diagram on one of the cliffs on Huashan, which he is said to have won as a sacred

mountain for Taoism by defeating the emperor in a game of chess. When I visited the mountain in 1999 there was still a pavilion marking the spot where the game took place.

The text is cultural, as opposed to martial, in the sense that it is concerned with the development of the self in an attempt to harmonize with the cosmos. It was written by a member of the literati for members of the literati, but its metaphysics and cosmogony have a resonance today in a time of climate change.

The *Tai Chi Diagram Explanation*

Wu Chi yet Tai Chi
Tai Chi moves to produce Yang
Movement to the limit (Chi) then still
Stillness then produces Yin
Stillness to the limit then returns to movement.
One movement, one stillness
Each acts as the root of the other
And (they) divide into Yin and Yang.
The Two Principles (Liang Yi) are established
Yang changes with Yin and they unite to
produce water, fire, wood, metal and earth.
The five Qi spread smoothly
The four seasons proceed on their course.
The Five Elements as one are Yin and Yang.
Yin and Yang as one are Tai Chi.
The origin of Tai Chi is in Wu Chi.
Once the Five Elements are
produced, each has its character.

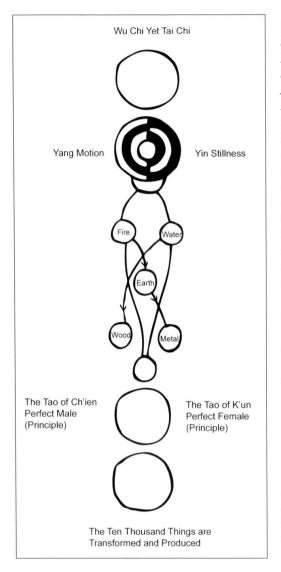

Wu Chi Yet Tai Chi

Yang Motion

Yin Stillness

Fire

Water

Earth

Wood

Metal

The Tao of Ch'ien
Perfect Male
(Principle)

The Tao of K'un
Perfect Female
(Principle)

The Ten Thousand Things are
Transformed and Produced

Fig. 132 Tai Chi Diagram of Zhou Dun-yi.

The reality of Wu Chi and the essence of Two (the Two Principles) and Five (Five Elements) wondrously combine and coagulate. The Tao of Heaven (Qian) perfects the Male; the Tao of Earth (Kun) perfects the Female. The Two Qi react (copulate) and influence one another, transforming and giving birth to the 10,000 things.

The 10,000 things repeatedly give birth and transform without end. It is only Man who obtains its excellence and who is the most intelligent. After his form has been born, his spirit discovers knowledge. The five characters (of the Five Elements) are stimulated and move. Good and evil are distinguished and the 10,000 things come forth. Sages fix matters using Benevolence and Righteousness (Ren Yi), Centrality and Correctness (Zhong Zheng). They advocate stillness and establish the limit (Chi) for man Formerly, 'the virtue of sages was in harmony with Heaven and Earth. Their enlightenment in harmony with sun and moon. Their sequence of actions in harmony with the four seasons. Their good and bad fortune in harmony with demons and gods.' (Quote from Book of Changes) The superior man's good fortune is in cultivating (virtue); The misfortune of the small man is in his nature. So it is said in establishing the Tao of Heaven, we speak of Yin and Yang. In establishing the Tao of Earth, we speak of Yin and Yang. In establishing the Tao of Man, we speak of Benevolence and Righteousness. It is also said, 'If one returns to the origins of things, one knows what there is to say about life and death.' How great is the Yi (Yi Jing/I Ching – Book of Changes). It is then the most perfect.

Commentary

Chu Xi, the greatest of the Neo-Confucians, wrote a commentary, explaining how the text is represented in the Diagram. The upper-most circle represents:

Wu Chi yet Tai Chi
Tai Chi moves to produce Yang
Movement to the limit (Chi) then still
Stillness then produces Yin
Stillness to the limit then returns
to movement

In the second figure down, the small central circle has the same meaning as the upper-most circle, while the half black, half white concentric circles are the source of one another and represent:

One movement, one stillness
Each acts as the root of the other
And (they) divide into Yin and Yang
The Two Principles (Liang Yi)
are established.

Underneath this, the next figure represents the interaction of Yin and Yang in the produc-tion of the Five Elements, each of which has both Yin and Yang aspects, and each of which is a type of *Qi* or vital energy. The small circle below the elements represents again *Wu Chi*, in which the elements are unified.

The last two figures represent the same principle of *Wu Chi* yet Tai Chi. The fourth circle emphasizes the Tao of Heaven perfect-ing maleness (the Yang principle) and the Tao of Earth perfecting femaleness (the female principle), both of which return to *Wu Chi* yet Tai Chi. The fifth and final figure focuses on the production and transformation of the 10,000 things, which again return to *Wu Chi* yet Tai Chi.

The Tao of Heaven (Qian) perfects the Male;
the Tao of Earth (Kun) perfects the Female.
The Two Qi react (copulate) and
influence one another, transforming
and giving birth to the 10,000 things.

The 10,000 things repeatedly give
birth and transform without end.

This is the most direct reference to Inter-nal Alchemy in the text. It is also the reason behind the name of the Heaven and Earth sword form that I practise.

The term '*Zhong Zheng*' can be found in writings of the Complete Reality School of Taoism. In his *Tai Chi Diagram Explana-tion* Zhou Dun-yi wrote, 'Sages fix matters using... Centrality and Correctness (*Zhong Zheng*).' This is using the term in a moral sense. Almost four centuries before Christ, the mystical meditation guide 'Internal Train-ing (*Nei Ye*)' has 'Correct mind (*Zheng Xin*) at Centre (*Zhong*)': to meditate effectively the mind has to be centred. There are many other references to centrality and correctness in the book, which may well have influenced Chu. In turn *Zhong Zheng* in terms of body alignment and posture became one of the key concepts of the TCC Classics.

Classic 1, like Zhou's explanation, deals with duality, change and the Five Elements. The beginning of Classic 2 is a restatement of the beginning of Zhou's explanation, with a strong emphasis on movement and still-ness. It also mentions 10,000 transforma-tions. Classic 3 talks of change; of 'Cen-trality and Correctness'; of movement and stillness; and of Ultimate/Limitless softness. Classic 4 also mentions transformation, with movement and stillness, and Centrality and Correctness. Classic 5 covers harmony, moving and not moving and using circular force (this last perhaps influenced by the Diagram itself).

The same terminology was, and is, used in martial arts, in meditation and alchemy, and in moral philosophy. The same people were practising the same things. They used the same concepts of duality, centrality and harmony; coming from and returning to *Wu Chi* yet Tai Chi.

13 Wu – Martial: General Qi Ji-Guang's *Classic of Boxing*

In the *Ji Xiao Xin Shu* (*Analytical New Book*), General Qi Ji-guang (1528–87) deals with all manner of military matters, including deployment of troops, use of signals, armed and unarmed fighting. We are concerned with the bare-handed techniques in Chapter 14 of the book, which is generally referred to as the *Classic of Boxing* (*Chuan Ching*/*Quan Jing*).

The *Classic of Boxing* is difficult to analyse in that the text details attacks, defences and counterattacks, yet each technique is only illustrated by a solitary boxer holding a solitary posture, and it is not always easy to decode either postures or text.

Some authorities feel that soldiers had little need for skill in unarmed combat, as a warrior always had his weapon with him. But this is illogical, because weapons can be lost, broken, stolen, or difficult to use in a specific situation. Japan's greatest swordsman, Miyamoto Musashi (1584–1645), in his *Book of Five Rings*, talks about punching, barging and grappling the enemy during sword duels. As he killed more than sixty opponents in such duels, we can assume he is right. In the Heaven and Earth sword form that I practise, many techniques are designed to be used against multiple opponents; for immediacy of action it is necessary to lock, throw, sweep, push or strike one opponent as the other is attacking. It makes sense then for soldiers to know how to fight when unarmed. Military unarmed combat is not quite the same as police or civilian self-defence, where the final aim is not normally to kill.

According to martial arts historian and Chen stylist, Gu Liu-xin, the earliest version of this book still in existence dates from 1595, with eight of the thirty-two boxing postures and their text missing. Perhaps because of this, and because people like to change things, there is confusion and dispute over the correct sequence. The one given here is from my own copy of Qi's book, published by *Zhonghua Shuju* in 1996. The *Classic of Boxing* lists nineteen different schools of boxing from which the thirty-two techniques were drawn, though nobody seems to know which technique comes from where or from whom. Most authorities believe that the techniques were designed to be practised as a choreographed sequence or form, just as TCC and many other martial arts are practised today.

I possess a copy of another *Classic of Boxing*, attributed to Emperor Song Tai Zu (960–983), founder of the Song dynasty. This Classic illustrates and lists thirty-two postures similar to those found in the Qi Ji-guang version, but the boxer is dressed in Song rather than Ming dynasty garb. The sequence is somewhat different from Qi's, and only the posture names and the illustrations are given; there is no accompanying explanatory poem. Most Chinese martial arts historians consider Qi Ji-guang's version to be genuine, though the order of the postures and other details may have been changed at various points. It is most likely that there was a Song Tai Zu or other version from which it was copied, and Qi Ji-guang even refers to Song Tai Zu. However, I suspect my version of the Song Tai Zu *Classic of Boxing* to be a plausible later fabrication.

Chen TCC contains almost thirty of these techniques (or at least that number of techniques with similar names). This strongly suggests that Chen style is a hybrid system put together by copying techniques from the *Classic of Boxing* (themselves drawn from nineteen schools of boxing) and Shaolin techniques such as 'Buddha's Warrior Attendant Pounds Mortar'. That is a whole different book, however.

Like the TCC Classics, the texts accompanying the individual postures are mnemonic ditties that can be easily memorized. Throughout the book the nature of animals is used to aid understanding of the techniques: thus Ox is heavy, Tiger sudden and ferocious, and Monkey full of changes.

There are some TCC elements and concepts in the preamble to the *Classic of Boxing* with references to softness and change, but the emphasis is on direct fighting techniques for troops. Throws, locks, strikes, chops, punches, kicks and weapon techniques are all mentioned. Some additional techniques that exist in TCC are mentioned in the texts accompanying the thirty-two postures; these include 'Low Technique', 'Draw the Bow' and 'Tiger Embraces Head', although they are not illustrated. It is common practice for techniques to be hidden inside others.

Many illustrations shown and explanations given in the *Classic of Boxing* bear little relevance to TCC theory or practice – for example, 'Overhead Cannon Style; rush the opponent to terrify him…' smacks more of the approach of external martial arts with its emphasis on sudden attack.

Now that the TCC Classics have been illustrated and explained, it should be easier for the reader to understand the *Classic of Boxing*. In my translation of Qi's preface, my comments are in brackets. For the postures, my commentary follows each ditty.

The *Classic of Boxing*

The most important requirements of the Classic of Boxing:

These skills are not the exclusive preserve of soldiers. Those who have ability and energy to spare, can in martial practice use (these skills). However, most people cannot train or understand well, but so much for that. This is why this essay comes at the end of the book.

Boxing methods (quan fa) seem not to be designed as skills for war (as opposed to individual combat self defence). However, moving the hands and feet with diligent limbs and lower body serves as the first way to learn and enter the door of the art, which has been handed down from ancient times to later generations, so it belongs to one family (that is, one style).

When learning boxing, move the body freely in accordance with the method. Hand techniques should be smooth (presumably in defence) and sharp (presumably in attack) in application. Leg methods should be light (in movement) and firm (in stillness). Advance and retreat in harmony (Chinese military strategy of retreat in order to attack). The legs can fly and soar (when kicking/jumping/evading).

Also, the best quality is to fall and get up, invert (cartwheel/roll/handstand forwards/back/sideways) and insert (put in my technique by stepping/punching/kicking between opponent's guard/attacks/technique); and when you want to be ferocious (to use speed and power), use split, chop and uppercut fists. When you want to be fast, grasp in a lively manner (like an animal seizing its prey) when (the opponent) faces heaven (that is, follow up when the opponent falls). When you want to be soft, know how to match (the opponent) with oblique evasion.

Therefore, (I) picked out good points of various boxing (methods) and selected thirty-two techniques. The techniques succeed one another (are linked together as a form or in application). In encountering the enemy and achieving mastery over him, the changes are infinite, subtle and grand without limit, deep and difficult to understand and use. Ordinary people are unable to see even a chink. If you can understand a little, you are already divine.

There is a common saying: 'fist hit, not know' (opponent does not know how he has been hit because the attack was so fast and skilful). It is a peal of thunder so sudden that the opponent can't cover his ears (he is deafened (hit) before he can cover his ears (before he can protect himself)).

So it is said: 'no provocation, no fending off (if I understand striking I don't need self-defence), then there is only one time (I only need to hit him once); if he tries to ward off blows, then there are ten times' (if he knows how to fight and defend himself, I hit him ten times). If you study in depth and learn broadly, the more you think, the more successful you will be.

Boxing experts of former times and now, have the thirty-two techniques of Long Boxing (Chang Chuan) from the Emperor Tai Zu of the Song dynasty (AD960–976); also Six Steps Boxing, Monkey Boxing and Decoy Boxing. Each has the specialities of its famous techniques, yet the techniques are really alike except for small differences. Up to now, also the best of the best were the Wen Family Seventy-Two Movements Boxing, Thirty-Six Closing Locks, Twenty-Four Throws Pat Horse, Dodging Eight Times and Twelve Shorts (Distance Boxing).

Though Lu Hong's Eight Movements are hard, and do not attain the level of Cotton Zhang's (cotton (mian) – here, as in the TCC Classics, it means soft) Short Striking (close-quarter fighting), the legs of Li bantian from Shandong (bantian is probably a nickname: half heaven – half of Shandong province had heard of him); Eagle Claw Wang's holds (a reference to Qinna – seizing and holding), the throws of Thousand Falls Zhang, Zhang Bo-jing's striking, the staff method of the Shaolin Temple, and the Qingtian staff method simultaneously (Qingtian is a famous place for boxing); the Yang family spear method and Bazi Boxing and staff, all are now famous.

Though each has its strong points, however, in use there is an above but no below, or there is a below but no above (no one art contains everything). By using any of them it is possible to gain victory over others. However, this is leaning to one corner (relying too much on one skill or speciality). If we use the methods of each family of boxing (that is, mixed together) and moreover practise them, truly it is like the snake strategy of Chang Shan (the idea of head and tail and of one technique following another). If you attack the tail then the head responds; if you attack the body then the head and the tail mutually respond. This is called 'above and below complete' and there is nothing it cannot defeat.

Generally speaking, in boxing, pole, sabre, spear, pitchfork, rake, sword, halberd, bow, darts, double sickles and using the shield, everything first comes from boxing methods, moving the body and hands. Indeed, boxing is the origin of the martial arts.

Now we will illustrate the techniques and explain them in (mnemonic) formula, to make it easier for those who study in later times to understand the art. On obtaining the art, we must try the enemy. We should feel no shame in failure and no pride in victory. We should be diligent in practising it over a long period (that is, try and think, think and try). If we fear the enemy, it is because our skill is too basic. More fighting will certainly refine the art. There is an old saying, 'if the skill is high, then a man's courage is great.' This is true and not false.

When I held public office on Chusan Island, I had the chance to practise boxing at Liu Cao Tang. I somehow violated the rules. Then (people called it) ten hits (I was hit ten times). This was fantastic, as amid sticks, I was continuously hit; continuously poked with one method.

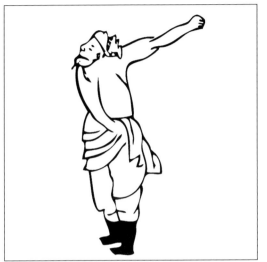

Fig. 133 Boxer 1.

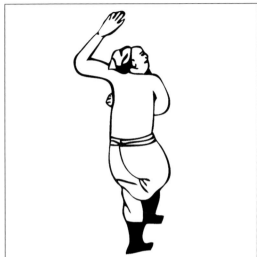

Fig. 134 Boxer 2.

Boxer 1
'Lazy Binding Clothes'; going
out the door technique
Change to Low/Next Technique,
quick steps Single Whip.
Face the enemy as if afraid of
nothing and go forward.
Empty yourself; eyes clear and hands ready.

Lan means 'lazy' and 'loose'/'relaxed'. In the Ming dynasty, men's clothes were folded across at the front and tied at the waist, but here they are tied lazily/loosely, preparatory to exercise. In the Qing dynasty, a long robe was worn with leg slits at the sides; this produced a tail, so the similar sounding 'Grasping Bird's Tail' was a reference to taking this tail up to exercise in comfort. Today some TCC styles use the name 'Lazy Binding Clothes'; others use 'Grasping Bird's Tail'. *Chu Men* – going out the door – refers to the first/beginning technique in a form.

Low/next technique – *Xia shi* is the same name as a TCC technique sometimes called 'Snake Creeps Down'. In TCC, *Xia shi* always follows Single Whip, but here the order is reversed.

The ditty instructs us not to look elsewhere, to focus and not be distracted.

Boxer 2
'Golden Cockerel on One
Leg', preparing to rise.
Pull back the leg(s) while giving
a crosswise punch.
Snatch with the Back, Reclining ox double fall.
After this my opponent incessantly
complains to high heaven.

'Golden Cockerel on One Leg' is a classical TCC technique. It requires the boxer to be erect and prepared to fight like a cockerel, maybe with one foot on tiptoe.

Line 3 describes the posture in the illustration, pulling back the right leg.

Line 4 seems to describe throwing the opponent over the back; using the bodyweight rather than the arms makes my attack heavy, as the weight of an ox and 'double fall' suggests I land on him to give a double impact.

117

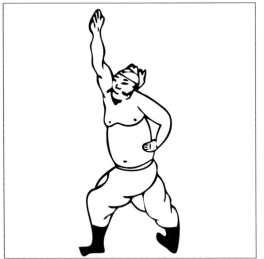

Fig. 135 Boxer 3.

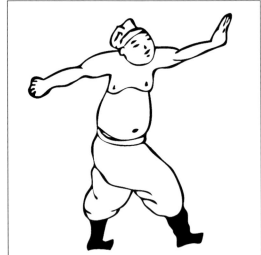

Fig. 136 Boxer 4.

Boxer 3
'Pat the Horse', handed down from Tai Zu.
The complete technique can be
more or less, and can change.
In advancing, attacking, retreating and
dodging, weakness becomes strength.
If you receive a short punch from
the enemy, this method is best.

'Pat the Horse' is a classical TCC technique, putting the opponent in a head or neck lock, but here the right arm position is exaggerated, which may suggest a palm strike before employing the lock. The technique comes from either Song Tai Zu (Song Supreme Founder, the first Song emperor) or from his time; he was known for his interest in Taoism. The first Jin emperor and the Hong Wu Emperor's temple were also called Tai Zu, but these are unlikely sources for the present reference.

It can be greater or smaller according to the circumstances – for example, inside or outside the opponent, distance, timing and the height of the opponent.

Boxer 4
'Bent Single Whip', Yellow
Flower advances urgently.
Open and lift his legs, left and right;
it is difficult for him to defend.
Snatch step and use the fist
continuously to chop the front.
Chen Xiang technique to push over Tai Shan

This is a second reference to Single Whip, a classical TCC technique. Yellow flower is a metaphor for virgin, so step like a virgin with closed legs when you advance, so the groin is protected.

Line 3 seems to suggest using sweeps and low kicks to disconcert the opponent and make him raise his legs.

Line 4 suggests a lunge step as in fencing – the drop step that the old American heavyweight, Jack Dempsey, refers to in his book. Some TCC exponents deny it can be done. They are correct: they can't do it.

In *Tai Chi Ancestors*, Professor Douglas Wile translates Chen Xiang as if it means something, but it is a proper name from

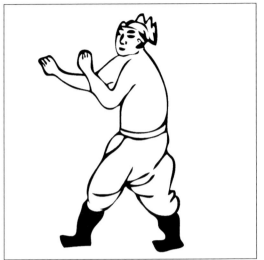

Fig. 137 Boxer 5.

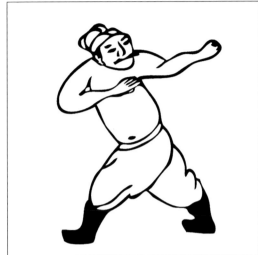

Fig. 138 Boxer 6.

Chinese mythology. Chen Xiang's mother had the sacred Taoist mountain of Tai Shan put on top of her and he lifted it off.

Boxer 5
'Seven Star Fists', hands and
legs are co-ordinated.
Step by step press, above and
below raise the cage
Even if he has fast hands and
feet like the wind,
I also can disturb and rush
him, chopping heavily.

There are a number of Seven Star techniques in TCC – sometimes the technique is used as a guard, sometimes it is applied with fists, sometimes with open hands. It can involve chopping, as here.

The second sentence advises us not to rush. The cage can be the arms, or a reference to Kung training, lifting heavy objects to strengthen the arms, such as carrying a cage, but more likely it refers to using a guard.

Disturbing the opponent suggests using feints to distract him before attacking.

Boxer 6
'Reverse Ride the Dragon',
pretend to lose and flee,
Entice the pursuer to enter, then
turn back and rush him.
No matter the strength and
ferocity of his powerful attacks,
How can he match my continuity,
which is like pearls strung
together or a cannon firing.

Line 2 suggests using the Chinese military strategy of 'retreat in order to attack'.

'Pearls strung together' is a metaphor for an attack with a barrage of techniques. *Pao*, meaning 'cannon', is one of the pieces in Chinese chess – and there is the *Pao Chui* form of Chen Style.

Boxer 7
'Hoist the leg' to entice him to
advance nonchalantly,

119

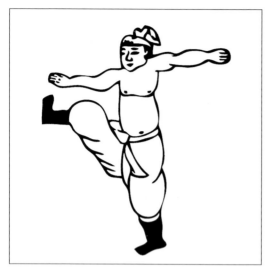

Fig. 139 Boxer 7.

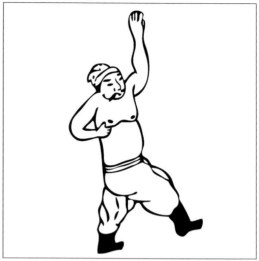

Fig. 140 Boxer 8.

Two changes of the legs and on
no account be merciful.
Matching this, above is one palm
and a whole heaven of stars.
Who dares to come again to compare skills.

He thinks I am vulnerable on one leg as I feint with a kick, and advances without thinking about it.

I put down one leg to attack with the other – a number of TCC techniques involve following one kick with another.

I then palm him so he falls and looks up to the stars.

Boxer 8
'Qiu and Liu technique', left
remove and right palm.
Stamp, taking a step and
connecting with the mind.
With heavy force, change boxing method,
Pat the Horse High while balanced.
Hit him once and cause his life to end.

Qiu and Liu are surnames, suggesting a master and student famous for a technique that was

then named after them. *Ban* – to remove/deflect – appears in the TCC technique *Ban Lan Chui* – 'Deflect Parry and Punch'.

After stamping, we step in and are prepared to follow up.

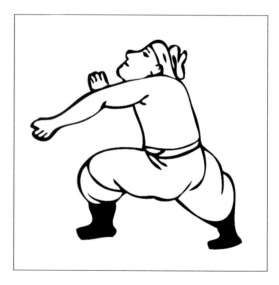

Fig. 141 Boxer 9.

'Heavy force' means using the whole body. This is a second reference to Pat the Horse, this time adding the term 'High'; as is the case in TCC, this suggests the head is the target. We use this technique when balanced.

Boxer 9
'Low Insert Technique' is to defeat fast legs.
Take the opportunity to advance, disturb
and get near/use Kao without separating.
Hook his leg and lock his arm,
not permitting him to leave.
Terrify him above and below he takes
a stumble.

I insert my low counter between his attacks/ guard/legs.

Line 2 means to go forwards, distract the opponent, and barge him in a continuous sequence. *Kao* is one of the Eight Forces in TCC, and means to hit with shoulder or body.

These moves are close together in distance and time, and knock the opponent down.

Boxer 10
'Lie in Ambush Technique'; bend
the bow awaiting the tiger.
If he rushes into the trap, he finds
it difficult to move away.
I then take the chance to
discharge continuous kicks.
When he receives the strikes, he
must be confused and afraid.

The body is bent in order to straighten; when the bow is bent, there is tension, and when released, power goes to upper and lower extremities and arms and legs. Tiger is the opponent. Draw/bend the bow to shoot the Tiger is a classical TCC technique based on a Zen story.

Boxer 11
'Throw Technique'; snatch/rush a
step, spread out and suspend.
Support the upper body and leg,
don't care if he knows.
Right horizontal, left uproot (cai) fast as flying.

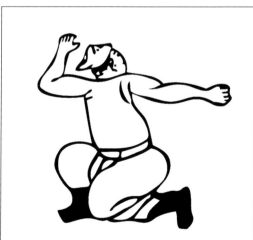

Fig. 142 Boxer 10.

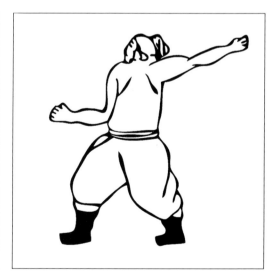

Fig. 143 Boxer 11.

In this posture one palm and he does
not know Heaven and Earth.

'Snatch step' is a lunge step as in fencing –
see Boxer 4. The Heaven Earth Sword has
consecutive techniques called 'Spread the
Sword' and 'Suspend the Sword', and I
suspect this is a similar technique, getting
around and behind an attack to unbalance
the opponent, then striking upwards.

Cai is using the hands to uproot the opponent, and not necessarily with one technique
– it could be as with TCC's 'Single Hand
Sweep Lotus Leg', grabbing the leg and neck
and flipping the opponent. The palm strike is
the coup de grâce.

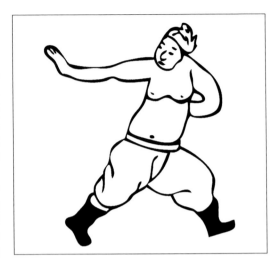

Fig. 145 Boxer 13.

Boxer 12
'Lift Forearm (Zhou) Technique'
defends against him using the foot.
When I intercept short range attacks,
I must know high and low.
Chop, push, hit and crush must
all be in conformity

Hands and feet are never in an urgent
situation in this technique.

Using the forearm – *Zhou* is one of eight
TCC methods of using force, and is used up
close, at which distance I must be ready for,
and prepared to use, high and low attacks. If

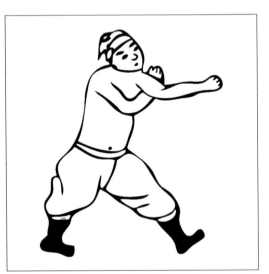

Fig. 144 Boxer 12.

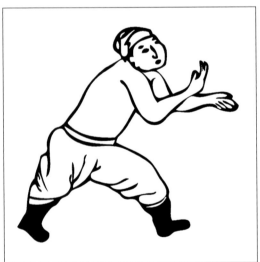

Fig. 146 Boxer 14.

I block his foot, he may use his hands, and vice versa: I am ready for anything.

Boxer 13

'With Sudden Steps' respond rapidly to changes.
Left and right, the legs rush the
opponent like pearls strung together.
No matter how strong his technique or whether
his hands are like wind and thunder.
How can he avoid my terrifying techniques
and my securing advantage by trickery.

The direction of the steps depends on the changes of the enemy. I attack him continuously with leg techniques, also employing feints so he can't defend himself.

Boxer 14

'Seize and Hold Technique';
seal the foot/feet in a loop
Left and right crush and press;
always four levels.
His directly oncoming fists fall
into my lively trap.
Even if he has quick legs, he cannot avoid this.

I use *Qinna* – seizing and holding, to set up a throw, lock or strike. Sealing the foot in a loop suggests catching a kick and putting on a foot lock or flipping the opponent. I change the direction of crushing or pressing force without him realizing it, while paying attention to the four levels of above head, below head, below waist and ground.

The trap is lively because it can change according to the situation.

Boxer 15

'Centralize Four Levels Technique', I push hard
I attack hard and advance, he with
fast legs finds it difficult to come.
Both my hands press on his single hand.
I use short strikes and familiar (techniques)
to deal smoothly (with the opponent).

The *Dantian* (a point just below the navel) is the centre of the four levels and the centre of gravity, so I sink to lower it and thus put more power into the push.

When I push I use two hands to control his one; this can be done by taking the

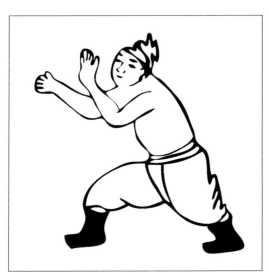

Fig. 147 Boxer 15.

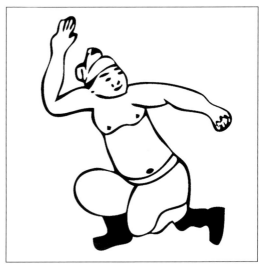

Fig. 148 Boxer 16.

opponent's arm from the outside and using it as a lever to control his body.

My training enables me to do this without thinking.

Boxer 16
'Crouching Tiger Technique', turn
halfway to play with legs.
If he approaches, I turn and rise
and use forearm to the front.
Seeing at once that he is not
 standing firmly,
To his rear I sweep with one kick
to separate what is clear.

I provoke his attack and catch his kick with a half turn. Next, I block his attack to the head. This, combined with the afore-mentioned 'catching the kick' is similar to the TCC technique 'Step Back to Ride the Tiger', and can also be used against the simultaneous attacks of two opponents.

Seeing his balance is disrupted, I sweep him. The character *ming* means 'clear' and is a combination of the characters for sun and moon. Separating what is clear suggests the opponent doesn't know what time of day it is after I have hit him.

Boxer 17
'High Four Levels Body Method'
with lively changes.
Left and right short; enter and exit as if flying
Force the enemy's hands and
feet so he is without ideas.
Thus I can conveniently kick and punch.

Here my short-range strikes are directed to the 'High Four Levels', the top of the head and between waist and head. My attacks are so rapid and varied that the opponent cannot cope.

Boxer 18
'Invert and Insert Technique', so I
don't need to ward off his attack.
Rely on quick legs to control him and to win.
Bend the back like a bow, and advance
without delay or hesitation.
Hit like an echo.

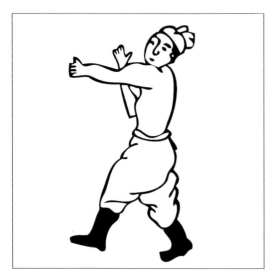

Fig. 149 Boxer 17.

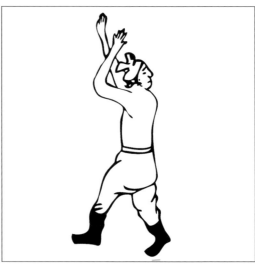

Fig. 150 Boxer 18.

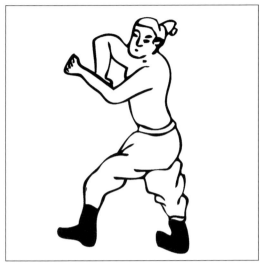

Fig. 151 Boxer 19.

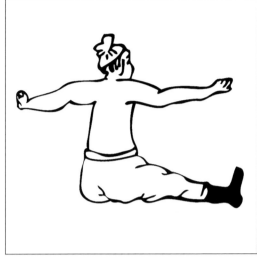

Fig. 152 Boxer 20.

This style is used to make defence into attack. Instead of blocking, I turn the opponent's technique over with a lock or flip, and insert a strike as he is defenceless.

'Bending the back like a bow' is similar to the imagery of TCC Classic 3, which says 'Accumulate the *Jin* (force) as if drawing a bow.'

'Echo' refers to the sound of fast and repeated impacts on the opponent.

Boxer 19
'Well Fence Four Levels', directly attack.
Cut the lower leg and hit the
opponent's head with the knee.
Rolling, pierce, chop, barge (Kao),
rub and (make) one hook.
I am like an iron general and he leaves.

The guard is the Well Fence, and we change from defence to sudden attack.

This cut blocks the opponent's kick, or is a sweep to his leg to set up a knee strike.

Six different attacks are then mentioned. Most likely these are alternative follow-up techniques to the four levels of the opponent after the knee strike. Rolling suggests

spinning to attack with the legs. *Kao* is one of the Eight Forces of TCC, and involves barging the opponent. Rub exists in a Shenxi style of *Pao Quan* and involves *Yin* (pull), *Bo* (push away) and *Kung* (control). In all things, I am firm like iron.

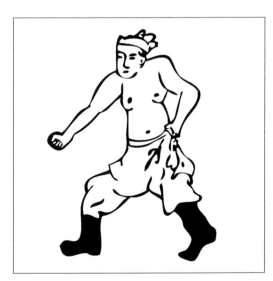

Fig. 153 Boxer 21.

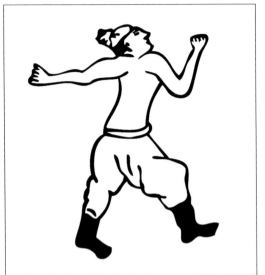

Fig. 154 Boxer 22.

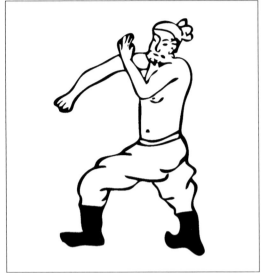

Fig. 155 Boxer 23.

Boxer 20
'Demon Kicks Leg'; catch up with
the opponent and I do it first.
Go forward, sweep his leg, turn the
body and use Hong Quan (red fist)
The back bends in order to
spring up and go forward.
Pierce the heart with Zhou & Kao. It
is so subtle it is difficult to describe.

I steal a march on the opponent, and rob
him before he robs me. The low sweep is the
'Demon Kicks Leg'. I use total body force
with forearm (*Zhou*) and barge (*Kao*), which
are two of the Eight Forces of TCC.

Boxer 21
'Point at Groin Technique' is a
method for male adults.
He finds it difficult to advance;
I want to face forward
Kick at his knees, with a spinning
jump/roll jump up to face him.
Hastily he turns his steps, I go
forward with short (range) Red
Fists (Hong Quan).

This is a punch to the groin, which exists in
Yang lineage TCC. Not surprisingly it is difficult for him to advance after this, so I kick,
spin, and follow up with short punches.

Boxer 22
'Beast Head Technique', like a
shield receiving an advance
Even if I encounter fast feet,
he will be disordered.
Low down he is startled, so high is chosen
and he finds it difficult to defend.
Intercept short (range) and uncover Red
(Fist) to rush against his upper level.

In the illustration the front hand is as if
holding a shield, something used for attack as
well as defence. This shield concept indicates
powerful total body movement; also animals
use their heads to attack. Thus if we butt the
opponent, the shield is the head.

I feint low, then hit high, possibly with said
headbutt, and at short range I punch him.

Boxer 23
'Spirit Fist' towards (opponent) insert low.

126

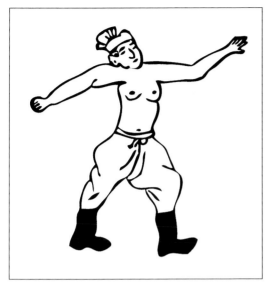

Fig. 156 Boxer 24.

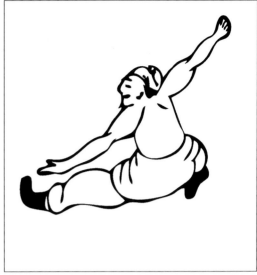

Fig. 157 Boxer 25.

Advance in a blaze of fire,
gathering the mind.
Change the actions/skills
according to the holds or kicks.
In raising the hands do not
show any mercy.

I suddenly step forwards with concentration
to insert low punch/es between the attempted
attacks of the opponent. I change my attacks
in accordance with his actions.

Boxer 24
'One Whip' horizontally,
chopping with the open hand.
Both legs advance to face the
opponent and injure him
Do not fear him though his strength
is harsh and his courage great.
I take the opportunity well to hit
him with magical power.

The posture shown does resemble TCC's
Single Whip, applications of which include
slaps and chops. This is the third reference to
Single Whip. I follow up with kicks.

Boxer 25
'Sparrow Earth Dragon', low basin leg method.
The front exposed and raised. Back foot
advances with Red Fists (Hong Quan).
He retreats, I, however, continue to hit him.

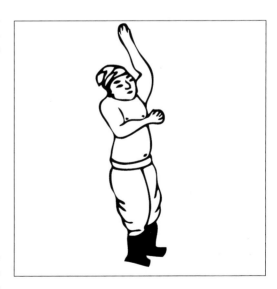

Fig. 158 Boxer 26.

Even if he uses short (range)
techniques to match me, it is in vain.

The posture shown resembles *Xia Shi* – 'Low Style/Snake Creeps Down' of TCC.

Possibly I am hitting him with double impact strikes. In 'Snake Creeps Down' if the opponent resists the takedown and steps back, we follow with a hit. As he is retreating there is no power in his attempted counters.

Boxer 26
'Facing Sun Hand', lean the body
to defend against his leg.
There is no space for him, lock and crowd
him; though a hero, he withdraws.
Inverted arrangement technique, and
I send him a searching foot.
Even a good teacher will thus
lose his reputation.

Here, I trap his arms and close him down, as I continue to pressurize him.

I turn back with a half step, the term used to search is *Tan* – one of the Eight Forces of

TCC sabre, and has the idea of scooping up from underneath: here it is a groin kick.

Boxer 27
'Wild Goose Wings', turn body and
advance with total body force.
Move with fast legs and
don't remain still.
Chase forwards and pierce
with the sole of the foot.
(I) Must add cut, chop,
push and Red (Fist).

We swing the arms like wings as we advance; the opponent expects more hands, so we use the leg as a surprise and follow it with some or all of the other techniques.

Boxer 28
'Ride Tiger Technique', move the
body, change legs and kick.
(I) Must move the legs without him realizing.
Left and right, sweep follows sweep.
His losing hands are easily
separated by my cutting blades.

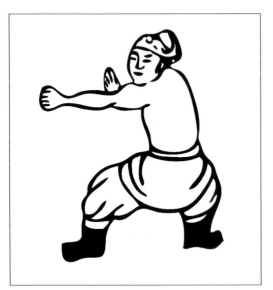

Fig. 159 Boxer 27.

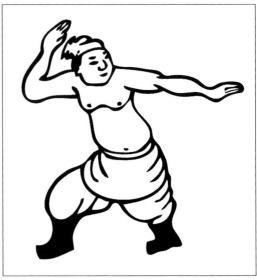

Fig. 160 Boxer 28.

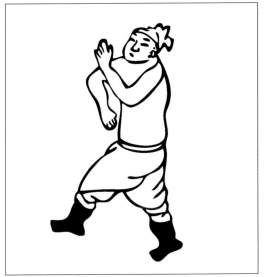

Fig. 161 Boxer 29.

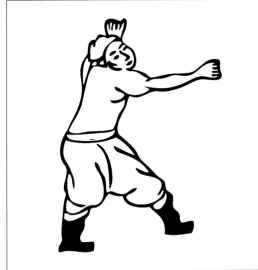

Fig. 162 Boxer 30.

'Step Back to Ride Tiger' is a classical TCC technique, also involving kicking. My follow-up sweeps make it impossible for him to defend.

Boxer 29
'Twist the Arms like the Luan', and
lunge forwards with a stamp.
Turn the palm to press down,
pluck and hit his heart.
Seize like an eagle laying hold of a
rabbit and firmly draw the bow.
The hands and feet must correspond.

The Luan is a phoenix-like bird. The character for 'twist' is the one appearing in TCC's 'Brush Knee Twist Step', so this indicates striking or defending with torsion, like the Luan does with its wings, for greater effect. Lunge is a drop step with the front foot.

I used 'press' for *Ban*, which is the same character as that meaning 'Deflect' in TCC technique 'Deflect, Parry, Punch'.

For the bird to rise after taking a rabbit, its wings need to open and flap; here the opponent is seized so he can be hit. A similar metaphor is used in TCC Classic 3, and also in TCC technique 'Draw Bow to Shoot Tiger'.

Boxer 30
'Aim at Head Cannon Technique';
rush the opponent to terrify him.
Advancing like a tiger, strike
directly with both fists.
He retreats and dodges, I again
bump and stamp him.
Even if not kicked down,
he will be disordered.

The Chen style may have borrowed the term 'Cannon' to refer to their Cannon Punch – *Pao Chui*. The technique is ferocious, fast and heavy, like a tiger. The stamp is likely to the knee joint, given the reference to being kicked down.

Boxer 31
'Smoothly use Luan Zhou', barge
(Kao) his body and move.

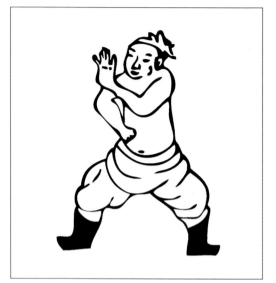

Fig. 163 Boxer 31.

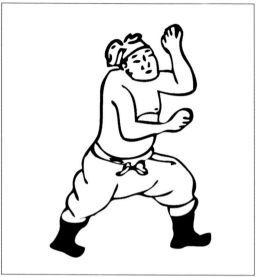

Fig. 164 Boxer 32.

Hit and roll quickly so it is
difficult for him to block.
Repeat the outside leg method
and rub control his back.
The body hit makes him fall, who
dares to stand in front of me?

The mythical Luan appears again, this time beating with its wings. Again the text mentions TCC tactics of *Zhou* – to strike with the forearm, and *Kao* – to lean or barge with the body or shoulder. This is followed by a spin.

Line 3 seems to suggest a trip using hand and foot in unison, as in TCC's 'Step Back Repulse Monkey'.

Boxer 32
'Flag and Drum Technique', left
and right crush and advance.
When I near him I use
horizontal chops with both hands.
With a circular step turning the body, I kick
the opponent and the opponent knows.
When Tiger Embraces Head, there
must be no door to hide.

The technique is like waving a flag or beating a drum. He knows there is no escape. 'Tiger Embraces Head' is a TCC technique using a punch or elbow strike to the opponent's head.

14 Conclusion: Tai Chi Chuan – Past, Present, Future

Deng Xiao-ping once remarked that Chinese history went from chaos to order and back to chaos. Similarly martial arts in general, and TCC in particular, seem to have gone from simplicity to complexity, but perhaps have not yet returned to simplicity. Before 1850 there seems to have been very little TCC around in China. We know that for at least a few decades before this date TCC was being practised at the Chen family village, but there is much dispute about the origins of TCC before that time. There may or may not also have been TCC on Wudang Mountain or elsewhere in that period.

In any case, Yang Lu-chan's departure for Beijing in 1852 effectively caused a split. His student, Wu Yu-xiang, went to Zhao-bao village, where he trained with Chen Qing-ping and supposedly learned all his secrets in a month. In the space of a few decades, and from what seems to have been one point of origin, there developed four different schools: Chen, Yang, Zhao-bao and Wu Yu-xiang. Many books follow the orthodox line, that there are five major styles of TCC; this may once have been the case, but for a long time now the situation has been much more complex, with a host of different influences taken in or out by every style to a greater or lesser degree.

Fourth generation Yang family head, Yang Zhen-duo, was interviewed many years ago when he first came to the West. He was asked about Fast Form and two person forms, and replied that such forms did not exist in Yang family TCC – yet these very forms are being taught by people who claim to be part of the Yang lineage. So far have things gone that the Yang family now practises a Cannon Punch (*Paochui*) form. It is traditional TCC in the sense that it is a new tradition.

The Chin Woo/Jing Wu (health and martial) Athletic Association was set up in Shanghai around 1910, and subsequently spread all over South East Asia. TCC of various styles was one of the arts taught, but there was no ritual initiation in Jing Wu. Instructors from Yang, Chen and Wu styles all taught in military academies in the nineteen-twenties and thirties. In a traditional Chinese martial arts school in the Far East, new disciples were, and are, expected to know and to earn their place in the hierarchy, particularly after ritual initiation. It is tacitly agreed that their conduct should follow the Confucian concepts of righteousness, benevolence and filial piety. Not surprisingly the Great Helmsman and the Chinese Communist party (Chicoms) did not regard this type of 'feudalism' with enthusiasm, although they expected to have it exhibited towards themselves. The Chicoms sent Wu Gong-zao, Wang Pei-sheng and many other masters to the Chinese gulag (*Lao Gai*) for this very reason. They did not spend their years in the gulag practising pushing hands.

The replacement in mainland China was gym or exercise Tai Chi (I do not use the term Chuan, as there was almost no martial element), where the movements were taught only as a choreographed exercise. China then was a place cut off from the outside world by the Bamboo Curtain. 'Feudal' ideas were vilified, and it was a mad world, where traffic lights signalled red for go and green for stop, where the corpulent Great Helmsman was surrounded by an army of adoring concubines, while the peasants starved in their fields as they made the 'Great Leap Forwards'. It was a country where *Shifu* (Cantonese *Sifu*) or teaching fathers could only be addressed as *Jiao Lian*, meaning 'coach' or 'trainer'. The TCC Classics were consigned to the dustbin of martial arts history, and chop-suey hybrid forms were created that had to be done in a precise way, which oftentimes conflicted with the principles of the said Classics.

TCC and the Present

This purely physical approach is quite inappropriate, and yet much TCC is of this type. These forms continue to be taught to this day, being changed a little every year or two by a committee, so those who practise them need to relearn if they are to be recognized as instructors, or in order to take part in competition.

The old boys who survived the gulag came back to a changed world, and inevitably their TCC had changed, too.

When I visited in 2004, there were more than 10,000 full-time students in ten Wushu schools at the Shaolin Temple, while Wushu schools covered the seventy-two peaks of Wudang Mountain like a rash. None existed when I first visited in 1984. Now it is again possible to use the term *Shifu* and to undergo *Bai Shi* (ritual initiation). In my visit to China in 2006 there were 50,000 students in eighty-three Wushu schools around Shaolin, and a five-star spa hotel complex with cultural village was being built on Wudang Mountain, involving the levelling of several peaks and

the destruction of Ming dynasty temples. What these people are doing is a physical art, but the practical, the therapeutic, the cultural, the Internal Alchemy approaches are noteworthy only for their absence.

Certain consequences have occurred as a result of oriental martial arts coming to the West. Since the sixties, a cabal of acupuncturists, tree-huggers, yoga and karate practitioners, hippies, mystics, experts in stress management and life coaching, and even academics, has attempted to hijack TCC and emasculate it by denying or ignoring the martial element. TCC came to the West in a series of waves. While the Bamboo Curtain was in place, Westerners went to Hong Kong, Singapore, Taiwan and Malaysia to learn TCC, and teachers from these places started to come to the West. From the late seventies, as China opened up, two-way traffic began, with students going to China and teachers coming to the West. The present situation is in flux.

Many practitioners believe that they are practising a traditional martial art, whether it be TCC or something else. In many ways this is far from true. In the twentieth century, various practitioners invented Tai Chi Ball, Tai Chi Ruler, Tai Chi Fan Form and other new practices such as performing Tai Chi to music, all now thought of by some as traditional. While TCC can be of great benefit to many people, it is time to reconnect with the Classics and reclaim the art – though some might think it is already too late. The TCC Classics are designed to be chanted and committed to memory, yet most practitioners (Chinese or otherwise) have never heard of the TCC Classics, far less are they aware of the truths therein. Never do they chant them. Classic 1 refers specifically to *Chang Chuan* (Long Boxing), comparing it to the great river, the Chang Jiang. Yet most people only practise short and simplified forms, a kind of nursery level TCC.

In any case, many Chinese characters have been wrongly or poorly translated. '*Jin*' is usually translated as 'energy', when it means 'trained force'. '*Sui*' is usually translated as 'yielding', when it means 'to follow'. '*Da Shou Ge*' is usually translated as 'The Song of Pushing Hands', when it literally means 'Striking Hands Song' and by extension 'Fighter's Song'. This leads to mistakes in practice and emphasis. Even when translations are correct, many of the cultural allusions and quotations from classical Chinese philosophy go over the heads of even most Chinese practitioners.

Many concepts are either misconstrued, or practitioners misunderstand how and when to use them. Thus, 'double-weighted' does not mean having the weight placed equally on each leg; 'suspended headtop' does not mean standing erect at all times; and using 'four taels to displace 1,000 catties' when defending against an attack does not prevent us from countering an opponent with considerable force. Yet many practitioners try to believe, and even to do, these ridiculous things.

The 'Song of Thirteen Tactics' states: 'To go through the gate and be led along the path, oral instruction is necessary; effort (*kung fu*) is unceasing; cultivate the method yourself.' Going to a TCC class once a week is not enough if you wish to progress beyond a basic level. This requires a personal relationship with a high level master, which includes private tuition followed by continuous self-development. Few are doing this: most just go to the nearest or cheapest class.

TCC and the Future

TCC has increased enormously in popularity since the 1970s, when I first started practising, and its popularity continues to increase, not least because of the interest generated by the 2008 Beijing Olympics.

However, detailed knowledge of traditional TCC practice is still rare – which is a great pity, as many of the old methods are fun to do, as well as being highly effective.

Now we have Tai Chi (the Chuan or boxing has disappeared!) for golf, for skiing, for tennis. There is Aqua Tai Chi, Nudist Tai Chi, Tai Chi for diabetes and many more. Normal TCC practice can do all the things that people running these programmes claim to do, as well as a lot more that, because of their 'fast food' approach, they fail to deliver. All this is really led by marketing, and those running the programmes are often better at commerce than at actual practice. A kind of antidote to this is the plethora of TCC events being held all over the world.

Research is now being carried out in relation to proprioception – the awareness of sensations beyond pure touch. Thanks to medical research, we know that every square centimetre of skin has about 200 pain receptors as well as fifteen pressure receptors, while each hand has around 17,000 touch receptors. We know also inner ear sensors can monitor head movements and make appropriate adjustments to the body's balance and posture. Numerous studies have shown TCC form practice to be a most effective way to improve balance and flexibility, as well as reducing blood pressure amongst the middle aged and elderly. At last, the medical establishment has embraced Tai Chi (again without the Chuan) as a way of preventing or treating problems such as heart conditions, arthritis, diabetes and the prevention of falls among the elderly. This is a huge area for further research, and can only increase our admiration for those men of genius who invented the Chinese internal martial arts.

The Classics in this book are a never-ending revelation, because perceptions will constantly change as knowledge increases. They influence our practice, which in turn affects our ability to understand them. The

Classics have a wider application than merely to teach us how to do TCC; many of the ideas can be used in daily life. In the end it is worth practising TCC for itself as a way of developing mind and body. For the modern martial artist it is an excellent way of learning new skills and enhancing old ones.

My old master sometimes referred to the martial arts as the 'world of truth and lies'. Lao Tzu said that 'beautiful words are not true, and true words are not beautiful'. I have tried in this book to separate true from false; the reader must judge to what extent I have succeeded. Practise well.

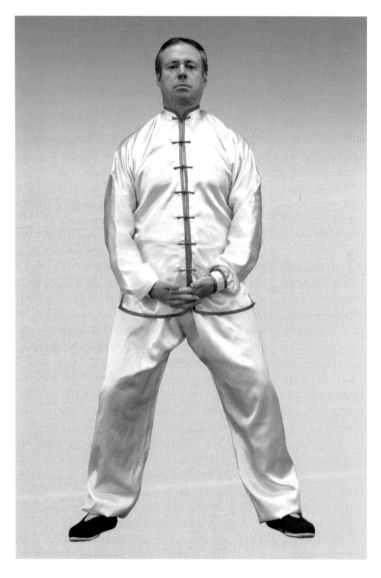

Author demonstrates a
Taoist Qigong posture.

Useful Websites and Addresses

With the advent of the internet there is a huge amount of information available about Tai Chi Chuan, most of it dross. A lot of people (mainly male) are writing and talking about TCC instead of doing it. I list below a few useful websites:

www.taichichuan.co.uk My own site with articles, reviews, training and instructor listings.

There is also a discussion group that covers topics relating to TCC, self-defence, therapeutics and other aspects of Chinese internal arts. The website has a large number of book reviews and book recommendations made by the author, and further reading in the form of the bibliography for this present volume is also posted. The author can be contacted at: dan_ptcci@hotmail.co.uk or write to 9 Ashfield Road, Southgate, London, N14 7LA, UK.

www.taichiunion.com Tai Chi Union for Great Britain official website with articles, events and instructor listings.

The TCUGB is the largest TCC organization in the UK. Membership is open to practitioners of Chinese internal arts, including TCC and Qigong. The TCUGB also publishes a quarterly full colour magazine full of reviews, articles and news about TCC from around the world.

www.tcfe.org Taijiquan and Qigong Federation for Europe official website with articles, events and member listings.

The TCFE organizes a bi-annual international forum and a bi-annual competition and festival of internal arts for its members.

www.bccma.com The British Council for Chinese Martial Arts is the Sports Council recognized governing body for Chinese martial arts, including TCC, in the UK. It is affiliated to the European Wushu Federation and to the International Wushu Federation, organizes competitions and provides insurance and licences for its members.

Glossary

I have mainly restricted the glossary to Chinese terms, and have rendered most of the Chinese expressions in modern Mandarin *Pinyin* romanization. In a few cases where the Cantonese or another Mandarin romanization system is more common in reference to a term, I have given that. Unfortunately a number of Chinese characters sound the same, but have quite different meanings, creating possible pitfalls for the non-Chinese reader. I've done my best in this glossary and in the text to give the major Chinese terminology and explanation in the hope that this is clearer than vague English translations for what are essentially technical terms.

An   Downward directed push/press.

Baduanjin Eight Pieces of Brocade. Chinese soft exercise for health, sometimes including techniques to stimulate the reproductive system.

Ba Gua/Pa Kua Eight Trigrams, consisting of the four cardinal points and four corners.

Ba Gua Zhang Eight Trigram Palm. Internal martial art based on Eight Trigrams.

Bai Shi   Ceremony of ritual initiation.

Bao Yi   To embrace the one (i.e. the *Tao*).

Bu   Footwork and stances.

Cai   Plucking or uprooting force.

Catty   Chinese unit of measure weighing more than 1lb.

Chan   School of Buddhism with heavy Chinese influences, better known in the West by its Japanese name of *Zen*.

Chang Chuan/Chang Quan Long Boxing. An alternative name for Tai Chi Chuan, as well as the name given to a hard style boxing form.

Chi/Qi Vital energy, including the air and breath (not the same Chi as in Tai Chi!).

Chi Kung/Qi Gong A method of training designed to increase the vital energy, for martial, health or meditative purposes, which can be hard or soft in nature.

Chien Trigram/hexagram representing Heaven and Supreme Yang.

Ching/Jing   Classic or Book.

Chuan/Quan Fist. By extension a system of fighting or boxing.

Da Lu Great sideways diversion. Popular name for famous pushing hands exercise, more properly known as Four Corners or Eight Gates Five Steps.

Dan Tian/Tan Tien Cinnabar field. Area just below the navel where Chinese alchemists considered internal energy was developed.

Dao   Sabre/broadsword.

Dao/Tao   Way or ways.

Diepu Fall and hit. Hitting an opponent when he has fallen, or making him fall by hitting.

Dim Mak/Dian Xue   Vital point attacks.

Fu Qi Spirit writing. The medium suspends a writing brush over a planchette filled with sand and invokes a spirit who communicates by tracing characters on the sand.

Gong/Kung Work/effort involving a degree of skill. In Chinese martial arts this usually refers to various types of conditioning training.

Hsing I/Xing Yi Chuan Form and Intent Boxing. One of the three major internal styles.

I Ching/Yi Jing Book/Classic of Change. A book of divination dating from before 1000BC.

Ji Straight push.

Jia Literally family or school.

Jian Sword.

Jiao Lian Trainer or coach.

Jin/Jing Force. We listen for our opponent's Jin, and redirect it with our own before discharging Jin at our opponent.

Jing Vital (often seminal) essence (not the same Jing as means force!).

Kao To lean. Applying force using the shoulder or back.

Kung Fu/Gongfu Skill/effort/workmanship. Often used by Cantonese speakers and Westerners to refer to Chinese boxing.

Kuoshu National Art. A general term for Chinese martial arts.

Lao Shi Old (i.e. venerable) teacher. Term of respect for teacher or master.

Li Strength.

Lie Using spiralling force.

Lu Diverting an oncoming force to the side and into emptiness.

Lun Theory/analect/discourse.

Men Ren Door Person. One who has become a disciple of a master.

Mian Chuan Cotton Boxing. Early name for Tai Chi Chuan.

Nei Dan Internal Alchemy.

Nei Jia Chuan Internal Family Boxing. Includes such arts as Tai Chi Chuan, Ba Gua Zhang and Xing Yi Chuan.

Nei Kung Internal Strength. More specifically a reference to the twenty-four Yin and Yang Internal Strength exercises.

Pai School of thought/boxing.

Pao Chui Cannon Punch. Name given to Chen Family Boxing and to their second form.

Peng Upwardly directed force, for example to divert a push upwards.

Qiang Spear.

Qinna Seizing and holding, often employing locking techniques.

Rou Soft.

San Shou Fighting techniques. Can also refer to choreographed two person forms, or to Chinese full contact fighting.

Shaolin Referring to the Buddhist temples of that name in Henan and Fujian provinces, and by extension to external martial arts identified with these temples.

Shen Spiritual energy.

Shi Style; for example, Hao Shi is Tai Chi Chuan in the style of Hao.

Shi San Shi Thirteen Postures/Tactics. An old name for Tai Chi Chuan.

Shuai Jiao Chinese wrestling.

Sifu/Shifu Teaching father. By extension any teacher or highly skilled person.

Song Relaxed.

Tael Chinese unit of weight, slightly more than an ounce.

Tai Chi/Taiji The Supreme Pole/Ultimate composed of Yin and Yang.

Tai Chi Chuan/Taijiquan A system of martial arts and exercise based on Yin and Yang.

Tao/Dao The Way or Ways to enlightenment or self-development followed by the Taoists.

Tao Te Ching Way and Virtue/Power Classic. Prime Taoist text credited to Lao Tzu (the Old Boy).

Tui Shou Pushing hands. Various partnered drills and exercises designed to improve skills such as close-quarter control of an opponent, evasion and co-ordination. Can also refer to free or competition pushing hands, where the object is to unbalance the opponent.

Tu Di Student or apprentice.

Wai Dan External alchemy. The use of medicines, and by extension a reference to external martial arts.

Wai Jia External family, referring to hard style martial arts.

Wu Chi/Ji No Ultimate. State before Tai Chi.

Wudang Referring to the mountain of that name.

Wu Shu Martial arts. Nowadays this Mandarin term has come to be used mainly in reference to the highly acrobatic and artistic modern martial arts routines.

Yang Active, male, positive principle representing strong, hard, external, bright, day, Heaven.

Yi The intent.

Yin Passive, female, negative principle representing gentle, soft, internal, dark, night, Earth.

Zhen Chuan True Transmission from a master to a disciple.

Zhen Ren True Person. Someone who has become a sage by Taoist methods.

Zhong Ding Centrally Fixed, corresponding to the element Earth.

Zhong Yong Doctrine of the Mean, text of the Confucians. Philosophical concept of acting only to the degree necessary, neither more nor less.

Zhong Zheng Centred and straight (though not necessarily upright).

Zhou Use of the forearm or elbow in defence or offence.

Zu Shi Founding teacher, for example Tai Chi Chuan putative founder, Chang San-feng.

Index